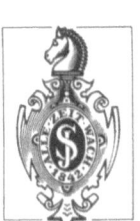

Jens Brange

Galenics of Insulin

The Physico-chemical and
Pharmaceutical Aspects of Insulin
and Insulin Preparations

With the Collaboration of
B. Skelbaek-Pedersen L. Langkjaer U. Damgaard
H. Ege S. Havelund L.G. Heding K.H. Jørgensen
J. Lykkeberg J. Markussen M. Pingel
E. Rasmussen

With 34 Figures and 20 Tables

Springer-Verlag Berlin Heidelberg GmbH

JENS BRANGE, M. Sc.
Novo Research Institute
Novo Allé
2880 Bagsvaerd, Denmark

ISBN 978-3-662-02528-4   ISBN 978-3-662-02526-0 (eBook)
DOI 10.1007/978-3-662-02526-0

© Springer-Verlag Berlin Heidelberg 1987

Originally published by Springer-Verlag Berlin Heidelberg New York in 1987.

The use of registered names, trademarks, etc. in this publication does not imply, even in the absence of a specific statement, that such names are exempt from the relevant protective laws and regulations and therefore free for general use.

Actrapid	Lente	Neusulin	Semilente
Humulin	Mixtard	NovoPen	Semitard
Initard	Monotard	Optisulin	Ultralente
Insulatard	Neulente	Protaphane	Ultratard
Lentard	Neuphane	Rapitard	Velosulin

Product liability: The publisher can give no guarantee for information about drug dosage and application thereof contained in this book. In every individual case the respective user must check its accuracy by consulting other pharmaceutical literature.

2127/3130-543210

Foreword

Galenical pharmacy or galenics is the science dealing with the production of drug substances from raw materials, the purity of such substances, their formulation into pharmaceutical preparations with the desired effects and safety in use, and the quality control, stability and storage of the preparations. The field has taken its name from the Greek physician Galen (131–201 A.D.), who had a profound influence on medicine for many centuries because he collected and systematized the medicinal knowledge of his time.

The discovery of insulin is attributed to Banting and Best who, in 1921, prepared an extract of the pancreas of the fetal calf and showed that the extract was capable of reducing the blood sugar level of a diabetic dog. This outstanding discovery gave rise to the rapid development of the manufacture of insulin of bovine and porcine origin. By 1925, two Danish manufacturers of insulin preparations were established; both have since been in the forefront of the development of insulin preparations, the latest achievement being the marketing of human insulin by Novo in 1982. The development of highly purified human insulin produced semisynthetically from porcine insulin or by DNA recombinant methods are significant contributions to safe and efficient insulin therapy.

Insulin is a protein which is destroyed in the gastrointestinal tract. It is therefore administered by subcutaneous injection using one of the many available preparations, which have different timing with respect to onset and duration of effect. The fact that the therapeutic index, i.e., the ratio between a lethal and an effective therapeutic dosis, is very low for insulin, together with the need for meal-related doses as well as a continuous basal supply, makes insulin an extremely challenging drug for pharmaceutical formulation. Improvements in bioavailability and investigation of alternative routes of administration of insulin, as well as a number of other proteins, represent major challenges to the pharmaceutical science today.

The present book covers all aspects of the galenics of insulin and will be most valuable to everyone aiming to know more about insulin and insulin preparations. This review will serve as a comprehensive reference source as to the properties of insulin and insulin preparations. In addition, it is a stimulating presentation of the many implications of insulin preparations and therapy.

Henning Gjelstrup Kristensen
Professor of Pharmacy
Royal Danish School of Pharmacy

Acknowledgements

The present monograph was originally intended for incorporation into a publication entitled *Subcutaneous Insulin Therapy,* which the editor had hoped to publish in 1983. The main aim was to compile a critical review of the subcutaneous insulin replacement therapy for patients with diabetes mellitus. The publication of the complete volume has been delayed considerably, and in late 1986 it was decided to update the present work and have it published as a single monograph. We are thankful to Professor Michael Berger and Springer-Verlag, who agreed to this solution.

The authors wish to thank E. Sørensen, M.Sc., for carrying out the immunogenicity studies, the prolongation test and biological potency estimations; A. R. Sørensen, M.Sc., for performing biological potency estimations; and Torsten Lauritzen, M.D., who was in charge of the absorption studies performed at Hvidøre Hospital, Klampenborg.

We also wish to acknowledge the skillful technical assistance of Lene Grønlund Andersen, Lene Bramsen, Lise Frank, Lone Jørgensen, Anne-Marie Kolstrup and Birgit Dræby Spon, the proficient assistance of Inger Jansson, who helped to prepare and assemble the manuscript and references, and the secretarial assistance of Mariann B. Andreasen and Dorte Schultz.

We are greatly indebted to Kathleen Larsen for her invaluable assistance in preparing the manuscript and to Dr. J. Schlichtkrull for his constructive criticism.

Table of Contents

A. Production of Bovine and Porcine Insulin

I. Introduction

Soon after the discovery of insulin by Banting and Best in 1921 processes were established for the manufacture of bovine and porcine insulin. Although these first insulins were very impure and caused undesirable side-effects they drastically improved the existence and the prospects of life for hundreds of thousands of diabetics. Later developments in insulin production leading to today's highly purified products have further improved the efficacy and safety of insulin therapy.

II. Physico-chemical Properties of Insulin Relevant to Production

That insulin is a protein was early recognised (Wintersteiner et al. 1928). The elucidation of its primary structure, however, was not established until 1955 after the extensive work of Sanger and coworkers, as reviewed by Sanger (1959). Fig. 1 shows the structure of porcine insulin. The bovine insulin molecule contains Ala (instead of Thr) and Val (instead of Ile) in positions 8 and 10 of the A-chain, respectively. Due to the size and structure of the molecule insulin may be called a polypeptide as well as a protein. The molecular weights are 5734 and 5778 for bovine and porcine insulin, respectively.

The insulin molecule contains many ionizable groups, due to 6 amino acid residues capable of attaining a positive charge and 10 amino acid residues capable of attaining a negative charge. Figure 2 shows the net charge of the insulin mol-

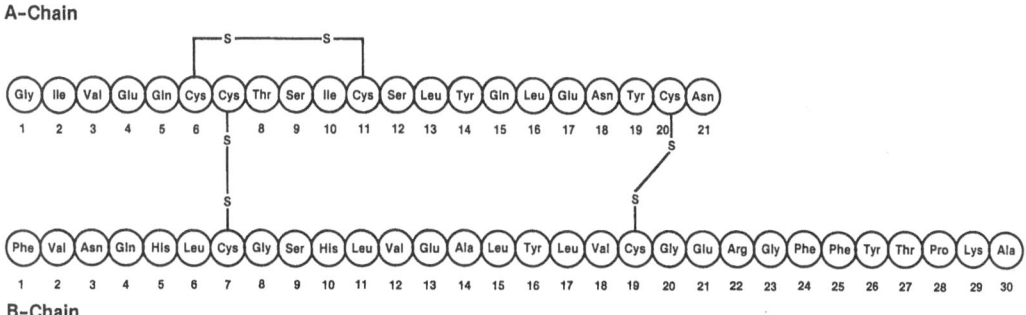

Fig. 1. The primary structure of porcine insulin

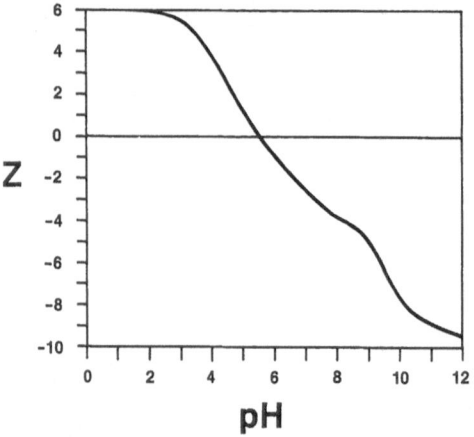

Fig. 2. The net charge Z of the insulin monomer as a function of pH. The following values of intrinsic pKa were used for the calculation: 7.2 (α-NH$_2$), 9.6 (ε-NH$_2$), 6.0 (imidazole group), 11.9 (guanidine group), 3.6 (α-COOH), 4.7 (γ-COOH) and 9.6 (phenolic groups)

ecule as a function of pH calculated on the basis of intrinsic pK values found by Tanford and Epstein (1954). The net charge is zero at pH 5.5, in good agreement with the electrophoretically determined isoelectric pH of 5.3–5.4 (Li 1954). One or more of the 6 amide groups in the insulin molecule may be lost by hydrolysis in solution (in particular at low pH, e.g. in 0.1 N HCl at 37 °C) leading to the formation of up to 6 carboxyl groups (Sundby 1962). Insulin degrades in alkaline medium (pH > 10) primarily due to its content of cystine residues (Cavallini et al. 1970). Insulin can be degraded by proteolytic enzymes, including those present in the pancreas, like trypsin, chymotrypsins and carboxypeptidases.

The solubility of insulin depends on a number of factors, such as the nature of the solvent, pH, temperature and the concentration of divalent metal ions and salts. In aqueous medium insulin can be precipitated at a pH interval around the isoelectric pH of 5.3–5.4 (Tanford and Epstein 1954). Bovine insulin precipitates easier than porcine insulin. At pH below 4 and above 7, both insulins are fairly soluble in the absence of Zn^{2+}. The precipitation zone is broadened towards higher pH values with increasing Zn^{2+} concentration (Schlichtkrull 1958). Insulin can be salted out at high concentrations of salts. Even at as low a concentration of insulin as 0.2 g/l a nearly complete precipitation takes place in 2 M NaCl at pH 2–3. Insulin is very soluble in homogenous mixtures of water and organic solvents, e.g. in 50–70% (v/v) ethanol. This uncommon property of a protein can be ascribed to the relatively low molecular weight of insulin and its relatively high content of hydrophobic amino acid residues (Val, Ile, Leu, Tyr, Phe). When the content of organic solvent in the mixture is very high the solubility of insulin decreases, depending on the kind of solvent, temperature, pH and salt content.

In aqueous solution insulin forms many kinds of association compounds due to non-covalent bondings; for a survey of these phenomena cf. C. II. 2. Addition of urea or organic solvents miscible with water, such as ethanol and acetic acid, counteracts such association. This effect is utilized in the chromatographic purification of insulin as described in A. IV.

Several crystal forms of insulin are known. Most important are the rhombohedral crystals composed of unit cells containing hexamers of insulin with 2 or

4 structural zinc atoms. The properties of these crystals and the kinetics of crystallization are summarized in C. II. 4. Two different crystallization methods are important for present day insulin production. The first method is based on crystallization at pH 6 in citrate buffer containing Zn^{2+} and 15% (v/v) acetone (Petersen 1945). The crystals formed contain two structural zinc atoms per hexamer of insulin (Schlichtkrull 1956a). The second method is based on crystallization at pH 5.5 in an acetate buffer containing 7% NaCl and 8–9 mg Zn^{2+} per gram of insulin. Using this method the crystals contain four structural zinc atoms per hexamer of insulin (Schlichtkrull 1958).

Detailed descriptions of the physico-chemical properties of insulin from a more general point of view, including insulins from other species than beef and pork, have been published in review form (Klostermeyer and Zahn 1971, Humbel et al. 1972, Schlichtkrull et al. 1975b).

III. Production of Crystalline Insulin

Until recently insulin for therapeutic use has been produced almost exclusively from bovine and porcine pancreas. According to a report from WHO (1980) there will be sufficient supplies of pancreas to meet requirements of insulin for the next decades.

The principles for the production of crude insulin have remained essentially unchanged throughout the past 40–50 years (Romans et al. 1940, Schlichtkrull et al. 1975b). Scott (1934) realized that insulin crystallizes in the presence of Zn^{2+}, which formed the basis for the subsequent introduction of crystallization as a step for purification of crude (amorphous) insulin. Figure 3 shows the main steps assumed to be representative for present day production of non-chromatographed insulin. The pancreata are deepfrozen (1) as soon as possible after slaughter in order to avoid enzymatic degradation of insulin. If kept below $-20\,°C$ during transport and storage (2) the processing of the glands can wait for several months without detectable loss of insulin. The content of insulin in pancreas is usually in the order of 0.02%. The use of acid ethanol/water for extraction (3, 4) ensures protection against enzymatic degradation, a high solubility of insulin and a low solubility of proteolytic enzymes, their precursors and many other proteins. The neutralization of the extract (5) renders possible the removal of substances which would otherwise create difficulties later on in the process. The evaporation step (6) serves the triple purpose of concentrating the extract, recovering ethanol and rendering possible the removal of fatty substances (mostly fatty acids and phospholipids) dissolved in the extract. In the salting-out step (7) insulin is separated from nonproteinaceous compounds and also from some foreign proteins and polypeptides. The salt-cake contains 15–20% insulin on the basis of total protein, depending on the kind of pancreas. The salting-out process may be repeated at a lower concentration of NaCl in order to obtain a further purification. The content of insulin in the precipitate formed at a pH-value close to the isoelectric point (8) is 50–60%. The first crystallization (9) is advantageously carried out in an acetone-Zn^{2+}-containing citrate buffer (cf. A. II). Insulin crystals with a very low content of glucagon are obtained by this method (Weitzel et al. 1953). The second

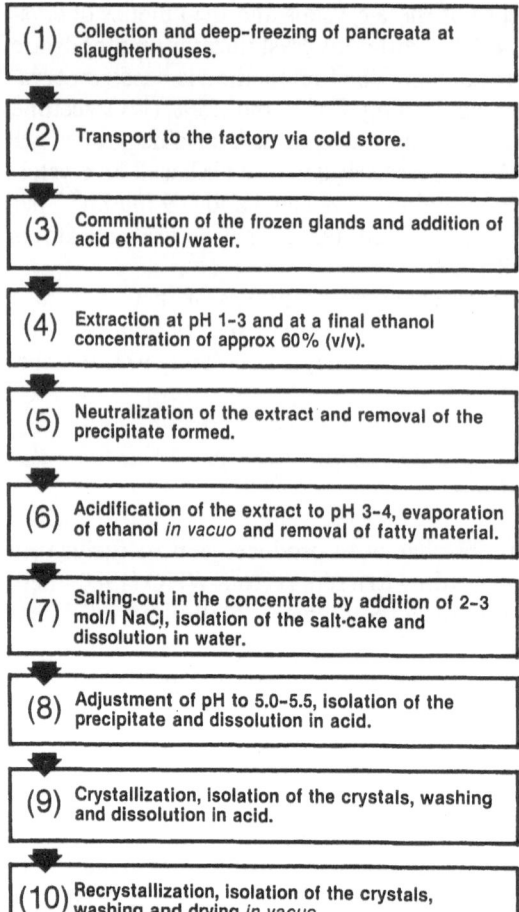

(1) Collection and deep–freezing of pancreata at slaughterhouses.

(2) Transport to the factory via cold store.

(3) Comminution of the frozen glands and addition of acid ethanol/water.

(4) Extraction at pH 1–3 and at a final ethanol concentration of approx 60% (v/v).

(5) Neutralization of the extract and removal of the precipitate formed.

(6) Acidification of the extract to pH 3–4, evaporation of ethanol *in vacuo* and removal of fatty material.

(7) Salting-out in the concentrate by addition of 2–3 mol/l NaCl, isolation of the salt-cake and dissolution in water.

(8) Adjustment of pH to 5.0–5.5, isolation of the precipitate and dissolution in acid.

(9) Crystallization, isolation of the crystals, washing and dissolution in acid.

(10) Recrystallization, isolation of the crystals, washing and drying *in vacuo*.

Fig. 3. Flow sheet of the production of porcine and bovine insulin from pancreas

crystallization (10) may be carried out by the acetate-salt method mentioned under A II. The recrystallization results in crystals with lower content of non-insulin-like contaminants. The purity of the twice crystallized insulin is 80–90% (content of insulin with the structure found by Sanger). If the insulin is not going to be purified by chromatographical methods, it is often subjected to further crystallizations before it is formulated into pharmaceutical preparations.

During the processing some insulin is inevitably lost. Other factors, however, also influence the yields, viz. species and race, age when slaughtered, the feeding and treatment of the animals in general, as well as the handling of the pancreata. The yields of crystalline insulin from one kilogram pancreas originating from beef cattle or from pigs are in the range of 100–200 mg. In dairy cattle the yields are somewhat below this range; whereas calf pancreas may yield as much as 400 mg of crystalline insulin per kg pancreas.

Reviews from a more general point of view on isolation of insulin (also concerning laboratory methods) have been published by Burgermeister et al. (1975) and Schlichtkrull (1975 b).

IV. Purification of Crystalline Insulin

After it became possible to crystallize insulin on a large scale, it was believed for some years that essentially pure insulin could at last be produced. Contributory to this assumption was the observation by Jorpes (1949) that insulin recrystallized up to 7 times was better tolerated by patients suffering from allergic reactions after treatment with conventional insulin. However, due to developments in analytical methods from the beginning of the 1950's until the late 1960's, it became increasingly clear that it was not justified to consider insulin purified solely by crystallization as a pure compound.

Heterogeneity of once crystallized or recrystallized insulin was revealed by a variety of methods, such as counter-current distribution (Harfenist and Craig 1952), partition chromatography (Carpenter 1958), anion- or cation-exchange chromatography (Thompson and O'Donnell 1960, Cole 1960), disc electrophoresis (Mirsky and Kawamura 1966) and gel filtration (Steiner 1967).

Identification of the detected non-insulin components, beyond the finding that some of them arose by deamidation of insulin, was not commenced until the work of Steiner and Oyer (1967), closely followed by the work of Steiner (1967), Chance et al. (1968), Schmidt and Arens (1968) and Steiner et al. (1968). Through the work of these researchers, it became clear that the b-component, revealed by gel filtration of crystalline insulin (cf. Fig. 4, B.I.2), was mainly composed of proinsulin, intermediates thereof and a non-convertible dimer of insulin, whereas two of the bands seen in disc electrophoresis of crystalline insulin (cf. Fig. 5, B.I.3), were due to proinsulin and its intermediates, respectively.

The a-component seen by gel filtration of once crystallized insulin (Fig. 4, cf. B.I.2) is composed of a series of high molecular weight compounds with a small content of insulin-related material (Schlichtkrull et al. 1974). The content of a-component can be considerably reduced by recrystallization, whereas the b-component is only slightly reduced in this way. Insulin itself is present in the c-component, which contains, in addition, insulin-like components, revealed by disc electrophoresis (Schlichtkrull et al. 1972), such as monodesamido insulin and a mixture of monoarginine- and monoethyl insulins formed by hydrolysis, conversion of proinsulin and esterification of insulin during extraction, respectively.

The results of immunogenicity studies in rabbits provoked the hypothesis that insulin impurities, not the insulin itself, were responsible for the immunogenicity of recrystallized insulin in patients (Schlichtkrull et al. 1970). As a consequence it was found desirable to purify insulin on a large scale, so that it displayed only a single component when analysed by both disc electrophoresis and gel filtration. In order for insulin to fulfill these criteria a method was developed based on anion-exchange column chromatography in ethanolic solution (Jørgensen et al. 1970, Schlichtkrull et al. 1972). It was later found that the purified insulin contained approx. 500 ppm homologous Proinsulin-Like Immunoreactivity (PLI), which could be reduced to less than 1 ppm by an additional chromatography (Schlichtkrull 1974). A survey of the development is given in the paper by Jørgensen et al. (1982). The twice chromatographed insulin has been named monocomponent (MC) insulin (Novo). Another example of twice chromatographed insulin in production is single component (SC) insulin (Lilly), made by a combination of gel filtration in 1 M acetic acid and anion-exchange chromatography in 7 M urea (Chance et al. 1976). The porcine RI insulin (Nordisk Insulin-laboratorium) is a third example of twice chromatographed insulin.

A great part of the insulin produced today is only purified by a single chromatography aiming at removal of the a- and b-component of crystalline insulin. Examples are SP-insulin (Lilly), CR- and CS-insulins (Hoechst) and mono-pic insulin (Organon). Most insulins used in current therapy have been subjected to one or another form of chromatographical purification, although a number of manufacturers still produce insulin purified only by crystallization.

B. Characterization of Insulin

I. Purity

1. Introduction

Proper characterization of the purity of insulin requires a combination of analytical methods based on various principles (Jørgensen et al. 1982). The four most important analytical principles for the characterization of insulin with respect to purity are the now classical biochemical methods of *gel filtration* (fractionation by molecular size) and *disc electrophoresis* (fractionation mainly by charge) to which have been added the highly sensitive methods of *radioimmunoassay* (RIA) and, recently, the *high performance liquid chromatography* (HPLC) methods. Improved modifications of HPLC techniques are expected to replace gel filtration and disc electrophoresis in the future.

2. Gel Filtration

In 1967 it was shown by means of gel filtration that commercial insulin, purified solely by crystallization, contained impurities with a higher molecular weight than that of insulin (Steiner 1967). These impurities were later identified to be mainly proinsulin, proinsulin intermediates and a covalent insulin dimer (Steiner et al. 1968).

Since then several gel filtration systems for the analysis of insulin have been described (Rolando and Torroba 1972, Schlichtkrull et al. 1974, Fisher and Porter 1981). Common to nearly all methods is the use of Bio-Gel P-30 (Bio-Rad Laboratories) or Sephadex G-50 (Pharmacia Fine Chemicals) and 1–3 M acetic acid as eluent. In this medium insulin is fully dissociated. Figure 4 shows three examples of gel filtration chromatograms of porcine insulin. In once crystallized insulin three distinct peaks are seen (*a, b* and *c*).

The a-component comprises high molecular weight substances (MW > 25,000) derived from pancreatic tissue proteins. Its concentration is reduced by crystallizations, but small amounts are still present in 5 times crystallized insulin, since antibodies against a-component are detectable in nearly all patients treated with insulin of this purity. (Heding et al. 1980).

The b-component contains proinsulin and related substances, which are removed to only a slight extent by crystallizations.

Finally, the c-component comprises insulin and derivatives of insulin with practically the same molecular size (insulin ethyl ester, arginine insulin, deamidated insulin, etc.) (Schlichtkrull et al. 1974).

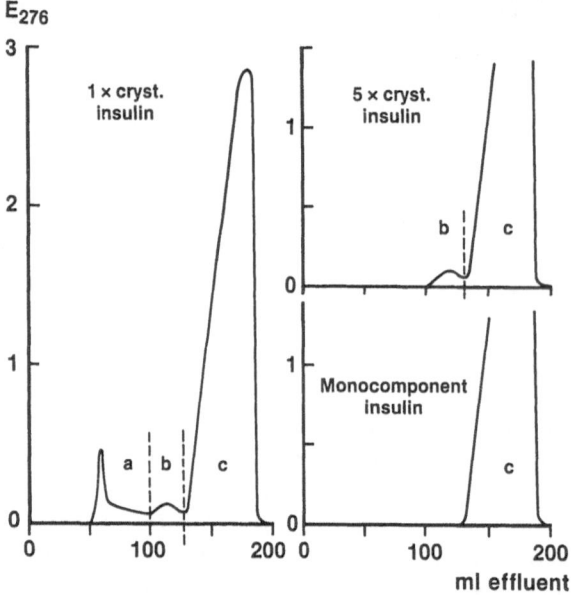

Fig. 4. Gel filtration of different porcine insulins on Bio-Gel P-30 (2.5 × 40 cm). Application of 100 mg of insulin dissolved in 1.5 ml of eluent. (Schlichtkrull et al. 1974)

Care should be taken when analysing insulin preparations by gel filtration to avoid possible misinterpretations due to the preservatives of the preparations (phenol, m-cresol or methylparaben). These substances absorb UV light strongly at the wavelength used for detection of insulin (275–280 nm) resulting in the largest peak of the chromatogram. An example of such a misinterpretation has been described by Schlichtkrull (1977a). Insulin isolated from preparations still contains traces of preservatives which will lead to peaks in the chromatograms. As the preservatives are of low molecular weight and tend to adsorb to the gel, they are eluted after the insulin peaks.

Gel filtration of insulin using HPLC technique (cf. B.I.5) has been described by Welinder (1980).

3. Disc Electrophoresis

Since the introduction of disc electrophoresis in polyacrylamide gels by Ornstein (1964) and Davis (1964), and Mirsky and Kawamura's (1966) subsequent application of this method for the analysis of insulin, it has been widely used for the characterization of insulin purity (Tjioe and Wacker 1972, Schlichtkrull et al. 1974, Krause and Beyer 1975, Kasama et al. 1980, Fisher and Porter 1981).

Although various electrophoretic systems are used by the different authors, they are all modifications of the original system by Davis and Ornstein operating at a slightly alkaline pH (8–9). Variations in acrylamide concentration, load per tube, content of dissociating agent (urea), and dye used for staining have been described. One of the most reproducible methods allows application of 100–200 µg of insulin per 5 × 50 mm tube containing 1 ml of gel (Schlichtkrull et al. 1974). At higher loads the insulin and monodesamido insulin are no longer distinguishable as two separate bands.

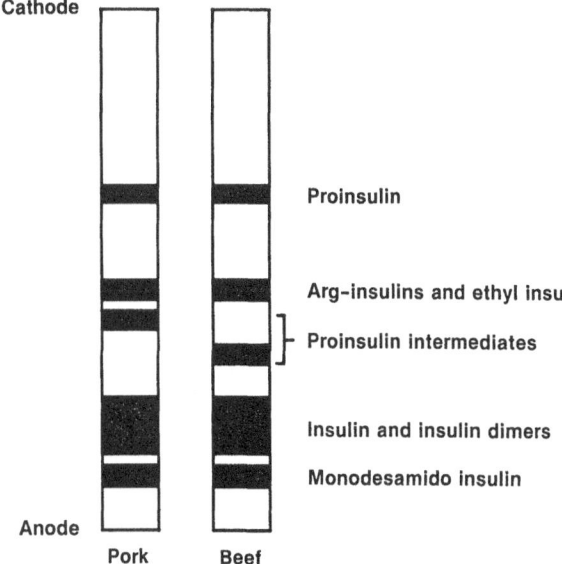

Fig. 5. Approximate positions
of protein components by disc
electrophoresis of recrystallized
insulin. As indicated the
positions of proinsulin
intermediates of pork and beef
insulin are a little different

Staining with Amidoschwarz in combination with diffusional destaining in 3% acetic acid is among the most reproducible methods for visualizing protein bands in polyacrylamide gels. Destaining by electrophoresis cannot be recommended, as weak bands may be removed by this method. A slightly more sensitive stain is Coomassie Brilliant Blue G 250, as used by Diezel et al. (1972), but meticulously standardized conditions during the staining procedure are required to obtain reproducible results. Therefore staining with Amidoschwarz is more convenient for routine purposes.

Figure 5 shows a schematic presentation of the position of the different protein bands resulting from disc electrophoresis of insulin purified solely by crystallizations. A rough quantification of the bands can be made by comparing with gels containing known amounts of the impurities added to monocomponent insulin. Another method is to compare with a series of gels to which varying amounts of insulin have been applied as a protein standard, as prescribed in the British Pharmacopoeia (1980).

Because of variation in ability to bind the dye and variation in band sharpness between the different impurities the latter method is less accurate than the former.

4. Radioimmunoassay (RIA)

Radioimmunochemical methods are by far the most sensitive used in the evaluation of insulin purity with a detection limit in the range of 1–500 ppb by weight (1 ppb $\simeq$ 1 part impurity in 10^9 parts of insulin). RIAs are two thousand to one million times more sensitive than the other methods described in this chapter (detection limits about 0.1%). RIAs have proved their great potential in detecting trace amounts in insulin of other polypeptide hormones originating from the extraction of the pancreatic glands.

Shortly after the discovery of proinsulin, the precursor of insulin, in 1968, it was found that commercial insulin preparations contained about 2% of proinsulin, and during the following years RIAs were developed for bovine and porcine proinsulin and C-peptide (Yip and Logothetopoulus 1969, Heding et al. 1974). The proinsulin RIA was the first of its kind used to evaluate insulin purity.

Proinsulin is composed of the insulin moiety and the connecting peptide. The sequence of the latter is highly variable between species. This allows the establishment of species specific proinsulin RIAs. Two methods have been used to eliminate interference from insulin:

a) The anti-proinsulin serum is passed through a column of immobilized insulin which removes insulin antibodies. The possibility of insulin interference is thus eliminated, and labelled proinsulin can be used as tracer (Yip and Logothetopoulos 1969, Aaby 1979).

b) The anti-proinsulin serum is used without pretreatment and insulin interference overcome by using a tracer that cannot be displaced by insulin, such as ^{125}I-Tyr-C-peptide (Heding et al. 1974). C-peptide contains no site for labelling with ^{125}I. Tyrosine is therefore coupled to the N-terminal amino acid of the C-peptide to yield Tyr-C-peptide, which is then labelled with ^{125}I (Markussen et al. 1970).

In addition to molecules containing the intact C-peptide moiety, the proinsulin RIAs may detect molecules containing fragments of the C-peptide. Thus, a better description of the material measured is given by the designation PLI (*Proinsulin-Like Immunoreactivity*), indicating that the trace contaminants in insulin may not only be proinsulin, but also other compounds with sequences partially identical to that of proinsulin.

The PLI in insulin is attributable to several impurities, consequently, standardization of reagents and methodology is necessary in order to obtain reproducible estimates of the PLI content in insulin (Damgaard and Kruse 1982, Kruse et al. 1984).

Shortly after a RIA for Glucagon-Like Immunoreactivity (GLI) became available analysis for GLI in insulin samples was introduced (Unger et al. 1970, Heding 1971). One of the major problems of this RIA is caused by the sensitivity of glucagon to proteolytic enzymes. Great care must be taken to avoid false estimates stemming from enzyme contamination leading to degradation of standard, tracer or the sample GLI. To minimize the problem a proteinase inhibitor, such as aprotinin, is added to the buffer to inhibit proteolytic degradation.

During the last decade new polypeptide hormones have been discovered to be present in the pancreas. This led to the application of additional RIAs for the characterization of insulin purity, namely for Pancreatic Polypeptide (PP) (Chance et al. 1979), somatostatin (Patel and Reichlin 1979, Tronier and Larsen 1982) and Vasoactive Intestinal Peptide (VIP) (Fahrenkrug and Schaffalizky de Muckadell 1977, Bloom 1979). Thus at least five different RIAs have been used for the characterization of insulin.

The level of some of the hormonal contaminants in insulin has been measured and found to vary greatly from brand to brand (Bloom et al. 1978, Fitz-Patrick and Patel 1981, Mizuno et al. 1980). Sutcliffe and Bristow (1984) reported that the

Table 1. Typical examples of contaminant contents (ppm) in twice crystallized and monocomponent insulin MC Novo

Contaminant	Twice crystallized insulin	Monocomponent insulin
PLI	20,000	$\leqslant 1$
GLI	45	$\leqslant 0.1$
PP	43	$\leqslant 0.01$
Somatostatin	1.4	$\leqslant 0.01$
VIP	0.3	$\leqslant 0.01$

PLI content in commercial bovine insulin formulations ranged from 0.23 to 4.8% for conventionally purified insulins, whereas the content in highly (chromatographically) purified bovine insulin varied between less than 1 ppm and 1160 ppm (0.1%). The contents of different hormone contaminants need not be correlated, as different purification methods may yield completely different compositions of the hormonal contamination (Jørgensen et al. 1982). Therefore it is unjustified to use a single contaminant as a common denominator of purity. A more comprehensive radioimmunochemical characterization should be used to evaluate purity.

Typical examples of the contaminant content of twice crystallized and monocomponent (MC) insulin Novo are shown in Table 1. It shows that careful application of modern purification technology can reduce the content of contaminating polypeptides in insulin to a level at or below the detection limit of the sensitive RIAs.

5. High Performance Liquid Chromatography (HPLC)

The most recent method for the analysis of insulin is HPLC. In particular the reverse phase mode of HPLC, with a nonpolar matrix as bed and a buffered mixture of water and organic solvent as eluent, has revolutionized polypeptide analysis by combining high selectivity and short time of analysis. Separation of bovine and porcine insulin was the first important application of HPLC in insulin chemistry (Biemond et al. 1979, Damgaard and Markussen 1979, Dinner and Lorenz 1979), followed by the separation of human insulin from the two other insulin species (Terabe et al. 1979). HPLC methods for separating several species including chicken, rabbit, sheep and horse have since been published (Ohta et al. 1983, Rivier and McClintock 1983). The introduction of HPLC means that high sensitivity species analysis of insulin preparations can now be performed in less than one hour.

The determination of monodesamido insulin formed by acid hydrolysis during extraction of insulin has traditionally been performed in a semiquantitative manner by disc gel electrophoresis (cf. B.I.3). A number of HPLC methods for the quantitation of monodesamido insulin have been published, and in most cases the species composition and monodesamido content can be determined in the same analysis (Szepesi and Gazdag 1981, Lloyd 1982). Lloyd and Corran (1982) have described an HPLC method capable of separating bovine, porcine and human insulin and their respective monodesamido derivatives in the same analysis. In contrast to the number of methods described for species analysis and determination of monodesamido insulin, few publications have described the use of HPLC for quantitation of impurities and insulin derivatives in insulin preparations. HPLC profiles of porcine insulin (Jørgensen et al. 1982, Welinder 1984), recombinant as well as semisynthetic human insulin (Chance et al. 1981a, Markussen et al. 1982) have appeared.

HPLC of conventional crystallized insulin has shown that insulin derivatives with virtually the same molecular weight as insulin, e.g. monoarginyl-insulin, monodesamido insulin and insulin ethylester, can be determined under isocratic conditions, i.e. using a constant eluent composition throughout the elution. Higher molecular weight compounds, such as proinsulin, proinsulin intermediates and covalent insulin dimers, need gradient elution with increasing elution strength in order to be analyzed with reasonable sensitivity in samples of insulin (Jørgensen et al. 1982). Recently, Welinder et al. (1986) have reviewed the literature concerning reversed-phase HPLC of insulin and investigated the influence of column geometry and eluent composition on resolution and recovery. Considering the increasing use of HPLC in insulin analysis during the last few years, little doubt remains that it will be one of the fundamental methods for species analysis and characterization of insulin purity in the future.

II. Standardization

1. Bioassay Methods

Several in vivo and in vitro bioassay methods for insulin have been developed. Only the in vivo bioassays based on the hypoglycemic effect of the insulin after injection into an experimental animal will be mentioned, since only these are recognized by health authorities for control of the biological potency of insulin for therapeutic use. The methods differ primarily in the species of animal employed, in the experimental design, and the procedure for handling the data.

During 1922–1926 bioassay methods for insulin were developed, based on the measurement of the hypoglycemic response in rabbits and the convulsive response in mice, in order to assess the potency of the hormone relative to an international standard. The 4th International Standard is soon to be replaced by a 5th generation of insulin standards of pure porcine, bovine and human insulin (WHO 1982). The classical bioassay methods, which contributed to the establishment of biometry, are still the basis for the pharmacopoeial methods for determination of insulin potency.

The rabbit blood sugar assay using a cross-over design was first suggested by Marks (1925). Since then there have been many publications recommending minor modifications to the original rabbit assay (Smith 1969).

Simultaneously with the development of the rabbit blood sugar assay, work was undertaken to utilize the insulin induced convulsions in mice first observed by Fraser (1923). Hemmingsen and Krogh (1926) and Trevan and Bock (1926) found that the percentage of mice responding increased with increasing dosage, and this led to the establishment of the theoretical basis for quantal response bioassays. Many studies have been carried out since of the precision and reproducibility of the mouse convulsion assay (Smith 1969, Stewart 1974).

Later, Eneroth and Aahlund (1968, 1970 a, b) have developed a mouse blood glucose twin cross-over assay.

Several papers have been published showing that the rabbit blood sugar assay, the mouse convulsion assay and the mouse blood glucose assay give essentially similar bioassay results (Miles et al. 1952, Bangham and Mussett 1959, Ashford et al. 1969, Bangham et al. 1978). However, an analysis of more than 500 rabbit blood sugar assays by new multivariate statistical methods showed that the potencies based on blood sugar responses ½, 1 and 2½ hours after the injection of pure porcine, bovine and human insulins relative to the present mixed species standard showed significant variation depending on the blood sampling times (Vølund et al. 1982, Pingel et al. 1985). Porcine and human insulin potencies decreased by 12% and 18%, respectively, from the ½-h to the 2½-h response, whereas bovine insulin potencies increased by 9%. Since the standard is approximately an even mixture of porcine and bovine insulin these results could be due to porcine and human insulin having a quicker onset and shorter duration of hypoglycemic effect than bovine insulin. This was confirmed in assays of porcine relative to bovine insulin and by direct comparison of mean blood sugar curves. It was concluded that the rabbit blood sugar assay is invalid when the test and standard insulin have a different species composition. Hence, pure species insulin standards are needed for this assay.

In the mouse convulsion assay no difference in the effect of porcine and bovine insulin has been demonstrated (Pingel et al. 1982). Thus this bioassay system can be used whether the test and standard preparation are of the same or of different insulin species.

2. Chemical Methods

Assessing the potency of insulins by a bioassay implies a certain risk of variation in the strength of the final insulin preparations. The use of a bioassay was mandatory in the years following the discovery of insulin, since the composition and purity of the insulins produced could vary considerably from batch to batch. Today, when insulins can be produced with a uniform and very high purity, it has become possible to reduce the potency variation between batches of pharmaceutical insulin preparations by calculating the potency of the insulin by accurate chemical methods of analysis, such as Kjeldahl nitrogen determination (Pingel et al. 1982) or HPLC (Kroeff and Chance 1982). Quantitation by HPLC of insulin and related substances in bulk insulin and in insulin preparations has been found to give an estimate of the potency that is in good agreement with that obtained by the rabbit blood sugar assay (Smith et al. 1985) and the mouse blood sugar assay (Fisher and Smith 1986). The HPLC method was found to reduce analysis time and to give more reproducible results. A bioassay may be used for control, and the potency estimate should be consistent with the estimate obtained by the chemical methods. The biological potency of MC insulin whether porcine, bovine or human has been found to be the same on a molar basis: $168 \cdot 10^6$ IU/mol corresponding to 184 IU/mg N (Pingel et al. 1982) determined by the mouse con-. vulsion assay.

III. Immunogenicity of Insulin

Awareness of immunological side-effects of insulin therapy became apparent during the late forties, and it was later established that virtually all insulin treated diabetics had insulin antibodies (Berson et al. 1956, Berson and Yalow 1959, 1964). In some patients the presence of high levels of antibodies caused severe insulin resistance due to the elimination of the insulin as antigen-antibody complexes (Berson and Yalow 1960). In other patients the antibodies were found to change the control of glycemia by firstly capturing the injected insulin, thereby reducing its biological effect, and later releasing it from the complexes, which could lead to hypoglycemia (Berson and Yalow 1960). These side-effects were thought to be inevitable until the introduction of the highly purified insulins in the early seventies.

Besides inducing insulin antibodies, insulin preparations containing detectable amounts of contaminants such as PP, VIP, glucagon and a-component, can induce antibodies against all these substances in insulin-treated diabetics (Bloom et al. 1979, Villalpando and Drash 1979, Heding et al. 1980). The biological significance of these antibodies is unknown. Radical elimination of the contaminants from the insulin has completely abolished the induction of such antibodies. When patients are transferred from conventional crystallized insulin to MC insulin a rapid decrease in the level of antibodies against the contaminants is observed (Heding et al. 1980). The mentioned antibodies all belong to the IgG class of immunoglobulin and bind and neutralize their antigen.

Antibodies of the IgE class specific for PP, a-component and insulin may also be induced by insulin preparations (Falholt et al. 1983). The IgE_I against insulin causes allergic manifestations. Insulin purified to MC specifications (Table 1) did not induce IgE_I, irrespective of the insulin species (Falholt 1982).

During the development of MC-insulin, aiming at reducing the formation of insulin antibodies (Schlichtkrull et al. 1970), an animal model was developed to control the various batches of insulin. The rabbit was found to be the most suitable species, as it develops insulin antibodies with similar capacity and affinity binding constants as do diabetic patients (Schlichtkrull et al. 1972). There is a considerable variation between the responses in rabbits to the same immunological stimulus but, irrespective of its shortcomings, the method is useful as a test for immunogenicity whenever new preparations or new technology for the production of insulin is introduced. In this rabbit model monocomponent porcine as well as human insulin exhibit non or very low antibody formation and the two insulin species cannot be distinguished from each other. In clinical trials, however, the immunogenicity of human insulin (cf. D.II) has, in several studies, been found to be lower than that of porcine insulin. After 6 months' treatment of 102 newly diagnosed diabetics with either porcine or human monocomponent insulin Schernthaner et al. (1983) found IgG insulin antibodies in only 14% of the patients treated with human insulin, but in 29% of those treated with porcine insulin. The antibody titres were also significantly lower in the patients treated with human compared to the patients who received porcine insulin. In a multi-centre trial Heding et al. (1984) compared the two insulin species in 135 newly diagnosed diabetic children and concluded that human monocomponent insulin has a lower immunogenicity than porcine insulin of the same purity during the first year of insulin treatment. In a long term study Luyckx and coworkers (1986) found that the percentage of patients who remained antibody-free after 12–21 months of treatment was 67–75% in the group treated with monocomponent human insulin and only 25–43% in the one receiving monocomponent porcine insulin, and the insulin antibody titres, when present, were lower in subjects treated with human insulin.

Velcovsky and Federlin (1984) also observed lower antibody concentrations in patients treated solely with human insulin compared to a group treated with porcine insulin and it was found that four diabetic patients with delayed-type allergy to animal insulin could be treated with human insulin without any problems. They concluded that the introduction of human insulins represents an important advance from the immunological point of view.

C. Insulin Preparations

I. Introduction

Banting and Best revolutionized diabetes therapy 60 years ago and extended the life expectancy of a young diabetic by decades. Since then the advances have been less dramatic, but important improvements and many refinements have emerged in the course of time.

The major achievements contributing to this progress are listed in Table 2.

Improvement in insulin purity – an essential element as regards character and quality of an insulin preparation – was the first challenge and has been a goal ever since, stimulated by the great advances in our knowledge of insulin from the work of Abel, Scott and Fisher, Jorpes, Sanger, Berson and Yalow, Schlichtkrull, Mirsky and Kawamura, Steiner and their coworkers, resulting in an ever increasing purity and the introduction of Actrapid – the first neutral insulin solution, MC-insulin – the first chromatographically purified insulin and, recently, human insulin.

Table 2. Major scientific achievements influencing the development and use of insulin preparations

1922	Isolation of insulin	Banting and Best
1926	Crystallization of insulin	Abel
1928	Insulin is a protein	Wintersteiner et al.
1934	Zinc insulin crystallization	Scott
1936	Protamine insulin	Hagedorn et al.
1936	Protamine zinc insulin	Scott and Fisher
1946	Isophane insulin (NPH)	Krayenbühl and Rosenberg
1949	Recrystallization reduces allergy	Jorpes
1951–52	Lente series	Hallas-Møller et al.
1955	Primary structure of insulin	Sanger et al.
1956	Radioimmunoassay	Berson, Yalow et al.
1958	4 Zn insulin crystallization	Schlichtkrull
1959	Biphasic insulin (Rapitard)	Schlichtkrull
1961	Neutral insulin solution (Actrapid)	Schlichtkrull et al.
1966	Heterogeneity (disc electrophoresis)	Mirsky and Kawamura
1967	Proinsulin	Steiner
1969	Tertiary structure	Hodgkin and co-workers (Adams et al.)
1970	Monocomponent insulin	Schlichtkrull et al.
1974	Continuous infusion	Pfeiffer et al., Albisser et al.
1979–81	Human insulin	Goeddel et al., Chance et al., Markussen
1980–82	Insulin pump implantation	Buchwald et al. Irsigler et al., Schade et al.

Numerous attempts were made to retard the subcutaneous absorption of insulin to spare the diabetics the chore and discomfort of multiple daily injections. Major milestones are the protamine- and protamine-zinc insulins, isophane (NPH) insulin, Lente insulins and Biphasic insulin. Crystallization of insulin and elucidation of the role of zinc for the association and structure of insulin have played an important role for this evolution and our understanding of insulin. Abel, Scott and Fisher, Schlichtkrull, and Hodgkin and their coworkers are the main contributors in this field.

A multitude of different insulin preparations are today available for the treatment of diabetics (cf. C. III and IV). The important characteristics from a pharmaceutical point of view, the analytical control, as well as the chemical and physicochemical properties relevant to their storage and use are discussed in various sections, however, it is not within the scope of the present chapter to go into details about the clinical usefulness of the various existing preparations.

Increasing awareness of the significance of strict metabolic control in the prevention of long-term complications of diabetes has somewhat paradoxically led to increasing use of the multiple daily injections of the early days of insulin therapy. Another approach is the use of insulin delivery systems initiated by the work of Pfeiffer et al. and Albisser et al.

The first implantations of such devices were performed in 1980–1981, a form of application which will require more stable insulin preparations. Before non-physiological additives are introduced for stabilization purposes thorough pharmacological and toxicological testing is mandatory. The same applies to the use of insulin analogues. (cf. C.X.II).

Alternative administration of insulin, such as rectal and nasal, as well as peroral, with absorption promoting agents or in liposomes, has been tried repeatedly with very limited success. New approaches like polymer implants and lectin-bound maltose insulins are being investigated (cf. C.XIII).

Despite 60 years' use insulin preparations are still undergoing development aiming at improving their therapeutic efficacy.

II. Pharmaceutical Chemistry

1. Insulin in Solution

The solubility of insulin depends on the species and purity of the insulin, the solvent, composition of the solvent, pH, zinc ion content, as well as the content of certain other divalent metal ions, ion strength and temperature.

In water insulin is practically insoluble at its isoelectric point of pH 5.4 (Fredericq and Neurath 1950), but is easily soluble at pH lower than 4. At neutral and alkaline reaction the solubility is strongly dependent on the concentration of zinc ions and on the species of insulin (Schlichtkrull 1958). Jeffrey et al. (1976) found the solubility of zinc-free bovine insulin at pH 7.0 to be 4.5–5 g/l, corresponding to approximately 125 IU/ml. Milthorpe et al. (1977) reported solubility of bovine zinc insulin crystals (2 Zn/hexamer) at pH 7.0 to be 0.9 g/l, corresponding to 24 IU/ml.

$$\text{Log} \left(\frac{\text{dissolved insulin}}{\text{total insulin}} \cdot 100 \right)$$

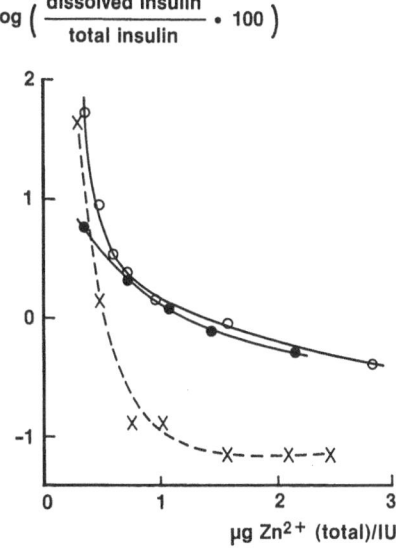

Fig. 6. Solubility of rhombohedral insulin crystals of different species and purity. Determination according to Schlichtkrull (1958) after 2 days at 20–25 °C in a medium containing 0.01 M sodium acetate, 0.01 M veronal (pH 7.4), 0.7% sodium chloride and 40 IU insulin/ml. Monocomponent porcine insulin ($\times$---$\times$) (Skelbæk-Pedersen, unpublished). Porcine (o—o) and bovine (●—●) insulin of conventional purity (Schlichtkrull 1958)

Using insulin purified only by crystallization, and having a total Zn^{2+} content of 0.37 µg/IU, the concentration of insulin in solution at pH 7.4 was found to be 2.4 IU/ml and 22 IU/ml for bovine and porcine insulin, respectively, at a total concentration of insulin (dissolved and suspended) of 40 IU/ml. At zinc ion concentrations above 1 µg/IU insulin is practically insoluble at neutral pH, irrespective of species (Schlichtkrull 1958, Schlichtkrull et al. 1975 a, b).

A reinvestigation of the solubility of porcine insulin of very high purity (MC-insulin), is shown in Fig. 6. In comparison with the earlier results it is evident that the removal of the impurities (proinsulin and derivatives, desamido insulins, etc.), as would be expected, lowered the solubility of the insulin.

IU/ml in solution

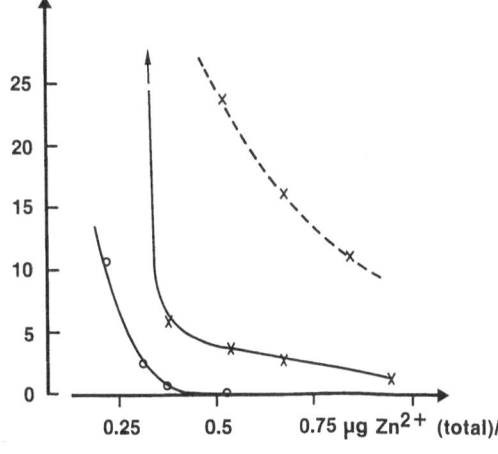

Fig. 7. Solubility of porcine MC insulin and porcine monodesamido-(A21)-insulin in neutral aqueous solution (pH 7) as a function of the total zinc content (Brange, unpublished). Insulin or monodesamido insulin in a total concentration of 40 IU/ml was dissolved followed by addition of the predetermined amount of zinc acetate, and allowed to stand for 3 days at 4 °C with frequent agitation. Monodesamido insulin (---), Insulin (——); with addition of methylparaben ($\times$——$\times$), without preservative (o—o)

Calcium ions have been observed to precipitate insulin in neutral solution, although not as effectively as Zn^{2+} (Emdin et al. 1980).

The solubility of insulin is also influenced by a variety of organic compounds. In neutral solution positively charged molecules may combine with negatively charged insulin molecules resulting in the precipitation of complexes. Thus, addition of basic proteins or peptides (cf. C.IV) or small amounts of cationic detergents (Birdi 1973) will decrease the solubility. The presence of glucose has been observed to augment the solubility of bovine insulin at pH 2 and 7 (Jeffrey 1974). Even the low concentrations of preservative present in the pharmaceutical preparations influence the solubility of insulin in neutral solution as shown in Fig. 7, which also illustrates that deamidation of insulin enhances the solubility.

The three-dimensional structure of insulin in solution is essentially identical to the structure of insulin in the rhombohedral zinc insulin crystals (cf. C.II.4) and assembly of monomers into dimers and hexamers (cf. C.II.2) does not alter the conformation of the monomeric unit in any important way (Bi et al. 1984, Hefford et al. 1986). The transformation from the 2 to 4 zinc structure (cf. C.II.4) has been found to occur in solution in a similar manner to that observed in the crystal (Williamson and Williams 1979, Ramesh and Bradbury 1986).

Dissolution of zinc insulin crystals is best carried out in acid solvent. Due to their zinc content the crystals dissolve very slowly at neutral and mildly alkaline reaction. Strongly basic solutions cannot be recommended because the disulfide bonds in insulin are very susceptible to degradation in alkaline medium.

2. Association of Insulin

Insulin exhibits a very complex association pattern in the crystalline state, as well as in solution. In solution it exists as an equilibrium mixture of monomers, dimers, tetramers, hexamers and, possibly, some higher associated states, dependent on concentration, pH, metal ions and salts. The monomeric insulin (bovine MW 5734) occurs in aqueous solution only at extremes of pH or in very diluted solutions. At pH 2 the monomer predominates only at concentrations below 0.5 g/l (Jeffrey and Coates 1966a). The dimer is the sole association species in the concentration range from 1 to 10 g/l when the ion strength is 0.05, but increased association up to an apparent molecular weight of about 25,000 can be observed when the ion strength is raised to 0.2 (Jeffrey and Coates 1966b).

At neutral reaction appreciable amounts of monomers only occur at insulin concentrations below 0.1 g/l (Frank et al. 1972). In diluted solutions (1–3 g/l) zinc-free insulin exists mainly as monomers at pH above 9 (Fredericq 1956).

The three-dimensional structure and the self-association of monomeric insulin into dimeric, tetrameric and hexameric molecules have been comprehensively reviewed by Blundell et al. (1972). When zinc or other divalent metal ions are present, the hexameric form prevails in neutral and moderately alkaline solutions. In solutions of bovine insulin at pH 7.0 with 2 zinc ions per 6 monomers of insulin, the hexamer comprises 75% or more of the total insulin at a concentration above 0.1 g/l (Milthorpe et al. 1977). Higher concentration of Zn^{2+} leads to association of two hexameric units (Fredericq 1956) and precipitation of the complex (Grant et al. 1972).

Calcium ions bind to zinc insulin hexamers at specific sites cross-linking three hexamers; this binding is most probably responsible for the decrease in solubility of zinc insulin at neutral pH in the presence of Ca^{2+} ions (Pitts et al. 1980).

It is mainly the nonpolar residues of the insulin monomer that are involved in the association into dimers and hexamers. The surface of the hexamer is therefore almost entirely polar (Blundell et al. 1972). About 40% of the surface of the monomers is buried in the hexamer (Renneboog-Squilbin et al. 1981). The receptor binding region of insulin has been found to include, in addition to more polar surface residues, many of the hydrophobic residues important to dimerization (Pullen et al. 1976). The molecular structure of the hexameric unit cell found in the crystal (Blundell et al. 1972) is assumed to be essentially the same as that observed in neutral solutions of zinc insulin (Frank et al. 1972, Goldman and Carpenter 1974, Strickland and Mercola 1976, Bi et al. 1984). Other studies, however, indicate that the crystal packing influences the 3-dimensional conformation (Renneboog-Squilbin et al. 1981, Bradbury et al. 1981). The average helix content has been found to decrease when the crystals are dissolved and conformational transition takes place when dissociation into monomeric insulin occurs in very dilute solutions (Pocker and Biswas 1980). From studies of the chemical reactivity of insulin at different concentrations it has been concluded that the monomeric unit has essentially the same conformation in its free and associated states (Kaplan et

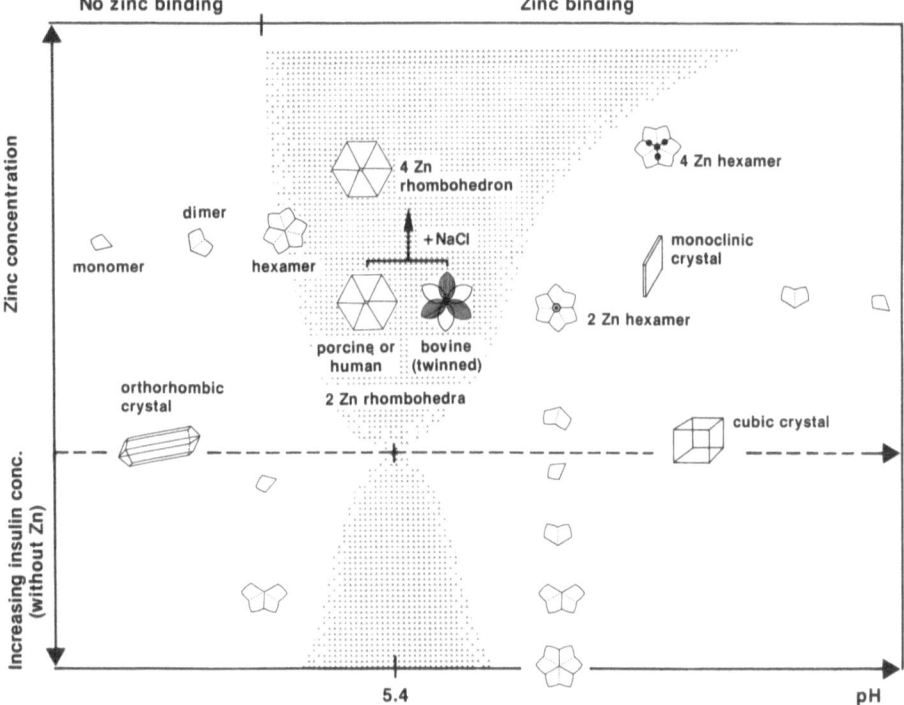

Fig. 8. Schematic diagram of the association and crystallization behaviour of insulin. The shaded area represents the insulin precipitation zone

al. 1984, Hefford et al. 1986), and Kaplan et al. pointed out that surface adsorption may have affected the data reported by Pocker and Biswas.

The association constant for the monomer-dimer equilibrium at pH 7.0 is $1.4–7.5 \times 10^5 \, M^{-1}$ (Pekar and Frank 1972, Jeffrey et al. 1976, Pocker and Biswas 1981, Strazza et al. 1985). Strazza et al. also showed that the dimerization properties are similar for bovine and porcine insulin and found that neither pH (pH 7 and pH 2) nor ion strength (0.1–0.01) influences the equilibrium constant significantly.

The value for the dimer-hexamer association constant at pH 7.0 for zinc free porcine insulin has been found to be $4 \times 10^8 \, M^{-2}$ (Pekar and Frank 1972). At pH 7.4 Holladay et al. (1977) found the value for zinc free bovine insulin to be $9 \times 10^9 \, M^{-2}$.

Pekar and Frank (1972) calculated the mole ratio of monomer to dimer at physiological concentrations (fasting state) to be about 8×10^5 to 1.

A schematic survey of the association behaviour of insulin under various conditions appears from Fig. 8.

3. Metal Ion Binding

The importance of zinc for the crystallization of insulin in the rhombohedral form was first recognized by Scott (1934) and later further explored by Schlichtkrull (1958), who found that the minimum zinc content necessary for crystallization was 2 atoms per hexamer.

Insulin is capable of binding large amounts of zinc either in the crystalline state or in solution in the slightly acid to the slightly alkaline range. At low pH insulin does not bind zinc (Cunningham et al. 1955, Schlichtkrull 1956a).

The interaction with zinc requires the formation of hexamers and is strongly pH-dependent. The content of bound zinc rises steeply when pH increases from 4.5 to 7.4 (Hallas-Møller et al. 1952, Schlichtkrull 1958) and is a function of the free zinc concentration (Cunningham et al. 1955). At pH 8.0 insulin is capable of binding 2.7 atoms of zinc per insulin monomer (Goldman and Carpenter 1974).

Two classes of binding sites with very different affinities for Zn^{2+} have been reported. In the pH-range 5 to 7 strong binding of two zinc atoms per hexamer of insulin occurs with an association constant of $10^5–10^6 \, M^{-1}$ at pH 7 to 8 (Summerell et al. 1965, Grant et al. 1972, Goldman and Carpenter 1974). The two zinc ions are hexacoordinate. Three ligands of each zinc ion are imidazolyl moieties of His (B10) from three monomers in different dimers (Adams et al. 1969, Bradbury et al. 1981). The remaining ligands are water molecules (Dunn et al. 1980) or small anions. Both metal binding sites are located on the trigonal symmetry axis, the metals serving to hold three dimers together in the hexamer (Brill and Venable 1968).

Above pH 7 an additional, weaker binding of zinc takes place with an apparent association constant of $10^3–10^4 \, M^{-1}$ at pH 8 (Goldman and Carpenter 1974). The involved binding sites have been found to include the α-amino groups in the insulin molecule (Marcker 1960, Frank et al. 1972). Chasteen et al. (1973), however, reported evidence that these sites are most likely the carboxyl groups of the glutamyl residues.

The porcine zinc-insulin complexes are soluble at neutral reaction when the zinc/insulin (hexameric) ratio is below 4, but at higher concentrations of zinc the solubility decreases (Finger et al. 1967) and at a ratio of 6 Zn^{2+}/hexamer complete precipitation of the insulin is observed (Grant et al. 1972).

A dynamic equilibrium exists between bound and free zinc ions, as all the zinc ions present in the crystalline structure are exchanged in the course of one hour (Schlichtkrull 1958).

During recent years it has been substantiated that the insulin hexamer in addition to the zinc binding sites also has three internal Ca^{2+} binding sites involving the Gln (B13) carboxylates (Sudmeier et al. 1981, Storm and Dunn 1985, Alameda et al. 1985). Such binding of calcium ions will neutralize the negative charges present on the six B13 glutamates in the central cavity of the hexamer, thus decreasing the solubility of the hexamer and facilitating the crystal formation in vivo in the β-cell granula of the pancreas.

4. Crystals and Crystallization

At least 6 different crystalline modifications of insulin have been discovered. The zinc-free orthorhombic crystals grown at acid pH by Ellenbogen (1949) and Sundby (1962) containing four dimers in the unit cell (Low 1952), the monoclinic crystals with 2 hexamers in the unit cell isolated by Schlichtkrull (1958) in neutral medium in the presence of zinc and phenol and further described by Harding et al. (1966) and Low and Chen (1969) and the zinc-free cubic crystals, obtained originally by Abel (1926), rediscovered by Schlichtkrull (1958) and structurally defined by Dodson et al. (1978) have never been used in therapeutic preparations (Fig. 9a–c).

The tetragonal crystals of protamine zinc insulin (Fig. 9 d) used in NPH preparations (Krayenbühl and Rosenberg 1946) contain, in addition to small amounts of protamine, at least 2 atoms of zinc and 20 molecules of phenol (m-cresol) per hexameric insulin. The protamine appears to occupy interstices in the structure between unusually packed hexamers (Hodgkin 1974).

The formation and shape of the rhombohedral zinc insulin crystals with 2 and 4 structural zinc atoms per hexameric unit of insulin have been extensively studied by Schlichtkrull (1957a, 1958). For review see Schlichtkrull et al. (1975a).

Schlichtkrull demonstrated that rhombohedral insulin crystals cannot be obtained without a content of zinc or certain other metal ions, thus finally elucidating the reasons for the previous difficulties in obtaining reproducible yields of insulin by crystallization. The minimum content of zinc ions necessary for crystallization is 2 atoms per hexamer, irrespective of pH of crystallization (pH 5.5–7.0) and species of insulin, indicating that the two atoms are an integral part of the crystal structure (Schlichtkrull 1956a). If, however, the amount of free zinc ions present in the crystallization medium prior to crystallization exceeds 6 atoms per hexamer of insulin the crystallization will be very slow or not take place at all.

When already formed the rhombohedral crystals are able to take up additional zinc ions, thus showing evidence for the existence of additional binding sites for zinc ions. The number of zinc atoms/hexamer increases to about 12 corresponding to about 2% zinc when pH is increased from 5 to 7.

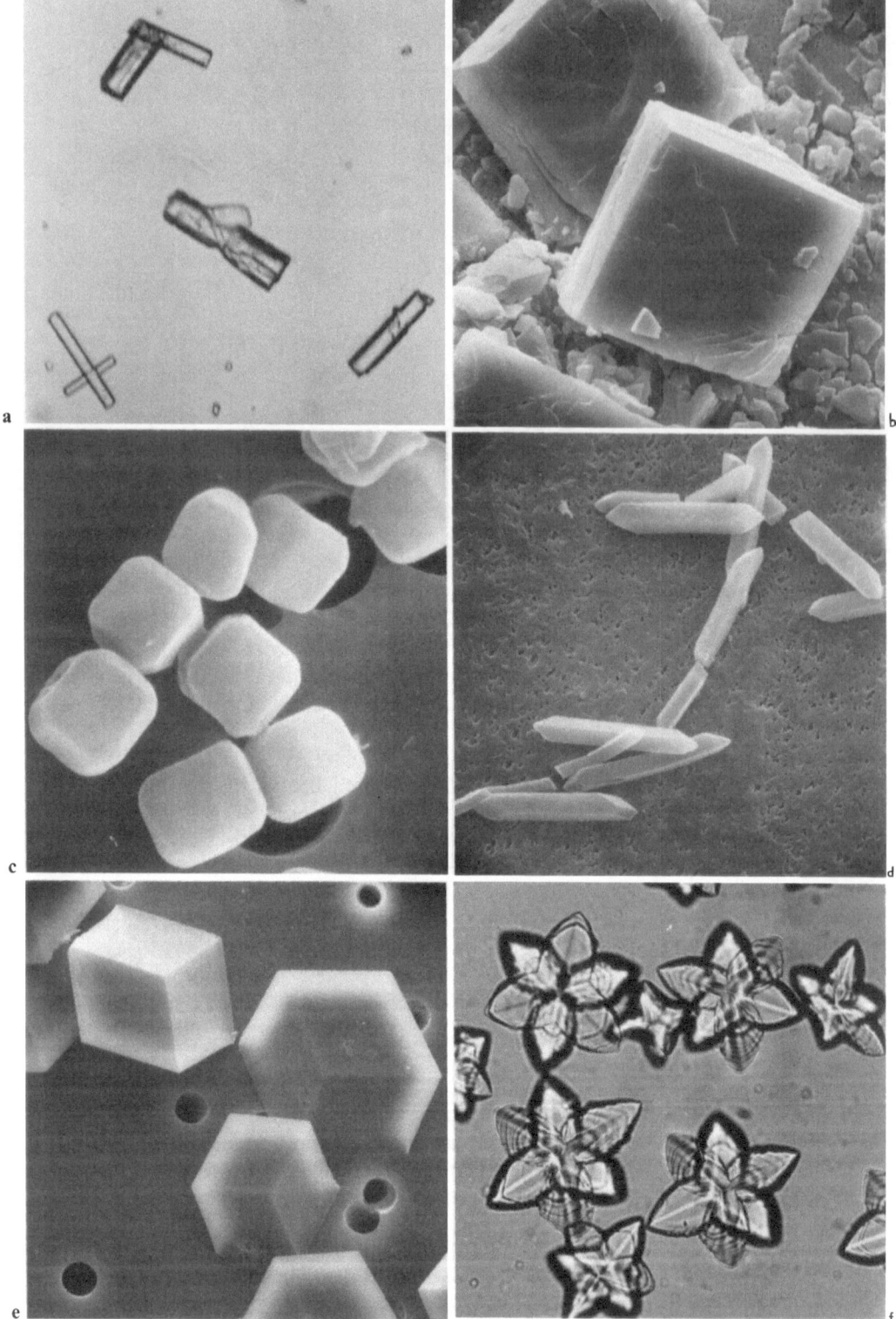

a b

c d

e f

The shape of the 2 zinc crystals with an internal rhombohedral structure varies with the species of insulin. Porcine and human insulins form geometrically perfect rhombohedra (Fig. 9 e), but bovine and ovine insulins have a tendency towards formation of distorted twin crystals often with a star-like appearance. (Fig. 9 f).

Another important factor determining the shape is the presence in the crystallization medium of halides or other insulin solubilizing agents. At sodium chloride concentrations above 6%, true rhombohedra are obtained irrespective of the species of insulin (Schlichtkrull 1956 b). Concurrently a steep rise in the structural amount of zinc ions from 2 to 4 atoms per hexamer is observed, the concentration of halide also being a relevant factor determining the shape (Schlichtkrull 1958, Schlichtkrull et al. 1957 a).

The three-dimensional arrangement of the atoms in rhombohedral 2 zinc insulin crystals has been elucidated by the extensive work by Adams et al. (1969), Blundell et al. (1971) and Dodson et al. (1979). The two zinc atoms are placed on the three-fold symmetry axis 9 Å above and 9 Å below the two-fold axes. The dimensions of the unit cells of 2 and 4 zinc insulin crystals are very similar with nearly identical lattice constants (Dodson et al. 1966), but surprisingly large structural differences in the protein conformation and organization of the zinc atoms were reported (Bentley et al. 1976, Chotia et al. 1983). In the 4 zinc crystals only one zinc ion appears on the three-fold axis and a considerable rearrangement of the first eight residues of the B-chain in 3 of the 6 monomers in the unit cell takes place. Despite the extensive structural differences a reversible interconversion of the two forms is possible simply by adding or removing chloride or other anions from the liquid surrounding the crystals. The transformation takes place within one to four hours – dependent on the temperature – with cracks appearing simultaneously in the crystals (Bentley et al. 1978). The 2 to 4 zinc conversion seems to be most efficient with anions high in the Hofmeister series (Williamson and Williams 1979, de Graaff et al. 1981).

The crystal structure of human insulin has been found to be nearly isomorphous to that of porcine insulin in the 2 zinc version (Chawdhury et al. 1983) as well as in the 4 zinc version (Smith et al. 1984).

The kinetics of insulin crystallization were investigated by Schlichtkrull (1957 c, d, e, 1958), who found that initial nucleation may take place on surrounding surfaces, e.g. the interface between liquid and air. Most of the crystal seeds are formed on the surface of existing crystals, the rate of self-nucleation being proportional to the product of the total surface of crystals and their growth rate. The growth of an insulin crystal is anisotropic, as insulin is only deposited on three of the six crystal faces, the rate being a simple power function of the concentration of insulin in solution.

Fig. 9. a Orthorhombic insulin crystals. × 380. b Monoclinic insulin crystals, × 1 800 (Scanning electron microscopy). c Cubic insulin crystals, × 4 500 (Scanning electron microscopy). d Tetragonal protamine zinc insulin (NPH) crystals, × 2 250 (Scanning electron microscopy). e Rhombohedral zinc insulin crystals, × 1 050 (Scanning electron microscopy). f Twinned, distorted rhombohedral beef insulin crystals ("stars"), × 380

In the preparation of pharmaceutical crystal suspensions monodisperse crystals are obtained by introducing a predetermined number of nuclei at the start of the crystallization (Schlichtkrull 1957 b). This seeding ensures that the crystals will be of the desired size and that the self-nucleation becomes almost insignificant.

In the crystallization of insulin intended for pharmaceutical suspensions a mixture is prepared containing approx. 1.5% of insulin, 7% of sodium chloride, 0.1 M of sodium acetate and a quantity of zinc ions adequate to give a total of 0.8–0.9% of zinc by weight of the insulin corresponding to 4 Zn atoms per hexamer of insulin. The pH is adjusted to 5.5 and the seeding crystals added. Initially almost all of the insulin is precipitated as amorphous particles. During the next hour some of the insulin gradually goes into solution, initiating the growth of the crystals, the fraction of which first increases rapidly and later more slowly. At the same time the concentration of dissolved insulin decreases, indicating that crystals grow from dissolved insulin (Fig. 10). The crystals formed are of the 4 Zn-insulin structure due to the high chloride concentration in the medium (7%).

In aqueous suspension the crystals contain 40–50% of water and have a porous structure allowing the diffusion of low molecular substances from the suspension medium into the crystal lattice.

Chemical compounds which interact with either the zinc ions or the insulin will change the crystallization pattern. The presence of phenol or its derivatives will produce non-rhombohedral insulin crystals, and zinc binding agents such as phosphate will hamper the crystallization.

The rate of crystallization is decreased by increasing the zinc content or the pH of the medium. At pH 7.4 and a total zinc ion concentration of 2 µg/IU the amorphous precipitate contains about 2.3% zinc and there will be no crystal formation for several years (Semilente).

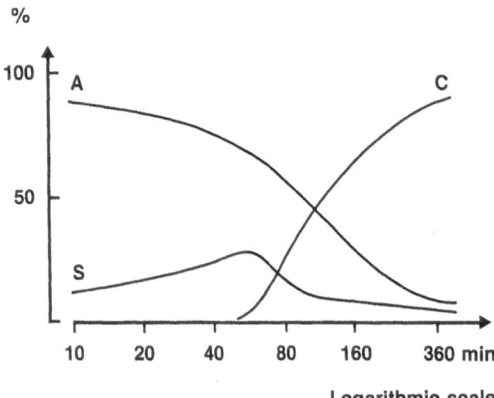

Fig. 10. Kinetics of Lente insulin crystallization. The curves represent the fraction of insulin in (*A*) amorphous, (*S*) dissolved and (*C*) crystalline state during the crystallization process. Insulin is crystallized from a mixture (pH 5.5) containing 400 IU/ml of insulin (bovine, recrystallized), 7% w/v of sodium chloride, 0.1 M sodium acetate and zinc chloride to give a total of 0.9% of zinc by weight of the insulin. (After Schlichtkrull 1957 c)

If, however, crystals formed at pH 5.5 are transferred to pH 7.4, the precipitate will remain crystalline (Ultralente). In the course of neutralization additional
zinc ions are captured to the same extent as in the amorphous insulin particles.

In the manufacture of the crystalline fraction of the pharmaceutical preparation Rapitard a transformation into the 2 zinc structure of the bovine 4 Zn crystal
is performed at pH 5.5 (cf. C.IV.4).

In the manufacture of Ultralente additional zinc ions are introduced parallel
with the pH-adjustment and a dilution of the sodium chloride concentration to
0.7%. Lange et al. (1979), studying porcine Ultralente crystals by electron and X-
ray diffraction, found a close resemblance to the 2 Zn insulin structure rather
than to the 4 Zn insulin structure.

Recently a new modification of the monoclinic crystal type of insulin has been
discovered (Brange, unpublished). Such crystals are easily formed when Ca^{2+} (or
Mg^{2+}, Ba^{2+}) is added up to a 3–5 mM concentration to neutral solutions of
Zn insulin containing 0.2% phenol (i.e. neutral regular insulin USP, cf. C.III.2).

X-ray studies on these Ca-insulin crystals have shown that they are closely
related to the monoclinic type without Ca^{2+} but distinct differences have been
observed (Dodson, personal communication). Experiments indicate that 5 Ca ions
per hexamer of insulin are bound to these crystals (Brange, unpublished).

5. Chemical Reactions

The chemical reactivity of the various functional groups in the molecule ob-
viously makes insulin susceptible to transformation. The variety of possible
chemical modifications have been summarized by Blundell et al. (1972) and
Schlichtkrull et al. (1975 b). More recent studies have indicated that some of the
amino groups of insulin are in a very reactive state at neutral pH values (Sheffer
and Kaplan 1979, Friesen 1979, Chan et al. 1981, Kaplan et al. 1984). Besides
Sheffer and Kaplan demonstrated that the amino groups will readily react with
CO_2 at physiological pH. A reaction between penicillin and the amino groups of
porcine insulin in neutral solution has been described by Corran and Waley
(1975).

Amaya-F. et al. (1976) studied the reaction between insulin and glucose in the
solid state and found that during 15 days at 37 °C and 70% relative humidity an
average of 1.4 hexose residues bind to the amino groups per molecule of insulin.
Addition of carbohydrates or glycerol (cf. C.XI.3) to neutral solutions of insulin
has been found to impair insulin chemical stability (Brange and Havelund
1983 b, Brange et al. 1982). Aldehyde impurities in the glycerol seem to be involved
in the chemical reactions seen when insulin is mixed with glycerol (Havelund,
unpublished).

The influence of heat, formulation, etc. on the different pharmaceutical
preparations is dealt with in section C.IX.

6. Mechanisms of Prolongation

The basic principle in prolonging the action of insulin is to delay the absorption
after subcutaneous injection by altering the solubility of the insulin at physiological pH. The different approaches relate to the following:

a) *Cationic organic compounds*, added to *acid solutions* of insulin. These will bind the insulin at the neutral reaction of tissue fluids making heavily soluble complexes. Examples of complexing agents are surfen and globin. The precipitates formed in vivo are more readily absorbed than preformed complexes.

b) *Neutral suspensions* of insulin combined with *basic proteins*. Examples are protamine zinc insulin (amorphous or crystalline variety) prepared with surplus protamine and Isophane (NPH) having a stoichiometric ratio between insulin and protamine.

c) *Neutral suspensions* of insulin complexed with small amounts of *zinc ions*. For further details cf. C.IV.3. Examples are: the Lente type preparations with 2 µg zinc per IU in U-40 preparations and crystals made of bovine insulin containing as little as 0.3 µg zinc per IU (Rapitard).

d) Alteration of the *physical state and size* of the suspended *insulin-zinc particles* entails variations in the duration of action. Small amorphous particles (Semilente) have a slightly slower effect than regular insulin, whereas crystalline particles (Ultralente) have a substantially more retarded effect, which again will vary with the size of the crystals (Fig. 11), emphasizing the importance of a uniform size distribution from batch to batch.

e) *Species of insulin* of the crystalline zinc insulin suspensions. The duration of action of the porcine crystals is somewhat shorter than that of the bovine variety (Fig. 11). An example is Lente (bovine crystal phase) versus Monotard (porcine crystal phase).

f) Chemical *derivation of insulin*. Hallas-Møller (1945) coupled the amino groups of insulin with phenylisocyanate (Iso-insulin). Schlichtkrull (1958) observed that special heat treatment of zinc insulin crystals at pH 5.5 (but not at pH 7) pro-

Residual fraction

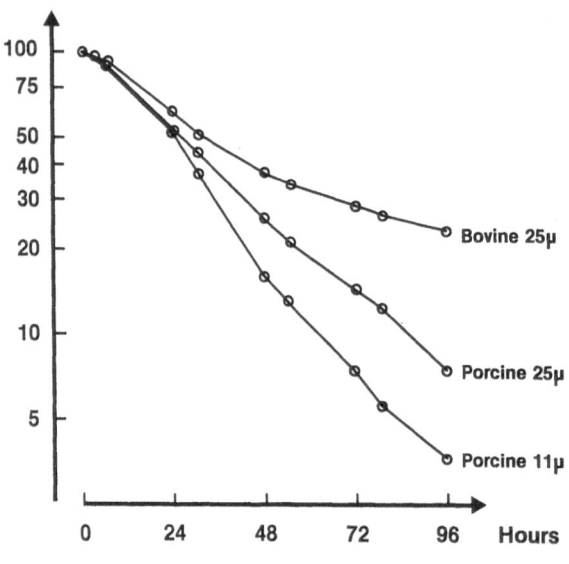

Fig. 11. The mean absorption course (method after Binder 1969) in six diabetics after subcutaneous injection of 12 IU ^{125}I-labelled Ultralente of different species and crystal size into the femoral region. (Lauritzen and Brange, unpublished)

duced a substantial enhancement of the retardation. No explanation was found at that time, but it has since become apparent that a chemical reaction between hexamers in the crystals takes place under those specific conditions, resulting in the formation of covalent dimers of insulin. The covalent link between monomers located in different hexamers will cross-link the hexamers within the crystals and thereby decrease the solubility of the crystals (Brange, unpubl.). Formation of only a few percent of dimer will cause a substantial change in solubility and, consequently, timing. A preparation of this type has been successfully used in treatment of streptozotocin diabetic rats (Rasch 1979).

III. Rapid-Acting Preparations

1. Introduction

In the early years of insulin manufacture only acid solutions of very impure insulin were available for diabetes therapy. A low pH was required to solubilize the foreign proteins and to protect the insulin from degradation by contaminating pancreatic enzymes. Removal of enzymes was achieved within the first decades of insulin production, but forty years elapsed before the overall purity of insulin was improved sufficiently to allow the manufacture of a neutral solution of insulin (Schlichtkrull et al. 1961, 1965).

The introduction of a retarded preparation in 1936 (Hagedorn et al., Scott and Fisher) ended the monopoly of the acid insulin solutions, but their great importance is reflected in the variety of synonyms (Table 3). Nowadays the term "regular insulin" designates a neutral insulin solution and is used in the following in this sense.

In recent years the increased awareness of the importance of strict metabolic control has resulted in multidose regimens featuring rapid acting neutral insulins as an essential part. The important aspects of mixing rapid-acting with intermediate and long-acting preparations are treated in section C.VIII.

In the future, regular insulins are likely to play a new role in therapy in connection with the increasing use of infusion pumps for insulin delivery. The need for more stable insulin solutions suitable for this application is discussed in section C.XI.

Table 3. Synonyms for acid solutions of insulin

Alt-(old) insulin	Quick-acting insulin
Clear insulin	Rapid-acting insulin
Crystalline insulin	Regular insulin
Crystalline zinc insulin	Short-acting insulin
Insulin injection	Soluble insulin
Normal insulin	Toronto insulin
Ordinary insulin	Unmodified insulin
Plain insulin	

2. Acid and Neutral Formulations

The formulation of commercially available, rapid-acting insulin solutions varies with respect to species, pH, zinc content, preservative, isotonic agent and buffering substance, if used. The compositions of different brands of neutral rapid-acting preparations are given in Table 4.

The neutral solutions may be better tolerated at the injection site. Besides they possess other advantages compared to the acid solutions. The chemical stability of neutral insulin is substantially better. The rates of deamidation during storage at 4 °C of two different acid formulations compared with a neutral solution are shown in Fig. 20 (cf. C.IX.2). A greater loss of potency is seen in the acid than in the neutral solutions during prolonged storage (Pingel and Vølund 1972). Another obvious advantage is their miscibility with the long-acting neutral insulin preparations without affecting the neutral pH of the mixture.

Andersen (1973) found that an acid solution gives rise to more insulin antibody formation than a neutral solution of the same batch of insulin.

Table 4. Composition of neutral regular insulin from various manufacturers (1983)

Manufacturer	Brand name	Species	Preservative	Isotonic agent	Other additives
BIM[a] (Wellcome, Boots, Evans) UK	Neusulin	Beef	Methylparaben	Sodium chloride	Sodium acetate
Connaught Canada	Insulin-Toronto	Beef	m-cresol	Glycerol	None
CSL[b] Australia	Nuralin	Pork	Methylparaben	Sodium chloride	Sodium acetate
Hoechst Germany	Optisulin CR	Beef (des-Phe^{B1})	Methylparaben	Sodium chloride	Sodium acetate
Lilly US	Regular Iletin I, II	Beef, pork, mixed	Phenol	Glycerol	None
	Humulin S	Human	m-cresol	Glycerol	None
Nordisk Denmark	Velosulin (Insulin Leo Neutral)	Pork	m-cresol	Glycerol	Sodium phosphate
Novo Denmark	Actrapid MC HM	Pork Human	Methylparaben	Sodium chloride	Sodium acetate
Novo Denmark	Actrapid MC HM	Pork, human	Phenol	Glycerol	None
Squibb US	Regular Insulin Injection USP	Pork	Phenol	Glycerol	None
Weddel UK	Hypurin Neutral	Beef	Phenol + m-cresol	Glycerol	Sodium phosphate

[a] British Insulin Manufacturers
[b] Commonwealth Serum Laboratories

Table 5. Viscosity and density at 20 °C of neutral regular insulins and corresponding media. Viscosity was measured with a Haake precision falling-sphere viscosimeter or a tube viscosimeter. Additives in the BP preparation: methylparaben 0.1%, sodium chloride 0.7% and sodium acetate 0.01 M; in the USP preparation: phenol 0.2% and glycerol 1.6%. (Skelbæk-Pedersen, unpublished)

	Insulin formulation					Distilled water (table values)
	BP			USP		
	Insulin concentration IU/ml			Insulin concentration IU/ml		
	0	40	80	0	500	
Viscosity (cp)	1.01	1.02	1.02	1.04	1.09	1.002
Density (g/ml)	1.005	1.006	1.006	1.003	1.008	0.998

The pH probably does not influence the rate of absorption of insulin solutions from the subcutaneous tissue (cf. C.III.4).

Stable neutral solutions of porcine zinc insulin containing 0.4% zinc (corresponding to approx. 2 Zn atoms per insulin hexamer) can be made in concentrations up to 500 IU/ml, which are used for treatment of patients with insulin resistance (Nathan et al. 1981). If zinc-free insulin is used it is possible to obtain a concentration of 5000 IU/ml in neutral medium.

The density and viscosity of different strengths and formulations of neutral solutions of zinc insulin are given in Table 5.

3. Manufacture

A neutral rapid-acting preparation may be made by dissolving the zinc insulin crystals in diluted hydrochloric acid at pH 3. The acid solution with an insulin concentration of about 4% is sterilized by filtration and mixed with solutions of the preservative, isotonic agent and, if included, the buffering agent. The solution is neutralized slowly with diluted alkali during which local excess of base is avoided by stirring continuously (cf. C.II.1.). The neutral solution is adjusted to the correct strength by addition of sterile water and filled aseptically into sterile vials.

4. Absorption

Binder et al. (1967) found neutral insulin to be absorbed faster from subcutis than an acid solution, however, Galloway et al. (1973) and Poulsen and Deckert (1976) found no difference in serum insulin concentration and hypoglycaemic activity, respectively, following subcutaneous injection of acid and neutral insulin. The discrepancy is possibly explained by the fact that the acid solution used by Binder contained five times as much zinc as the neutral solution. An acid insulin preparation will pass the iso-electric precipitation zone of insulin after injection, and a high zinc content will impede the redissolution of precipitated insulin and thereby delay the absorption. The high zinc content of acid solutions was found

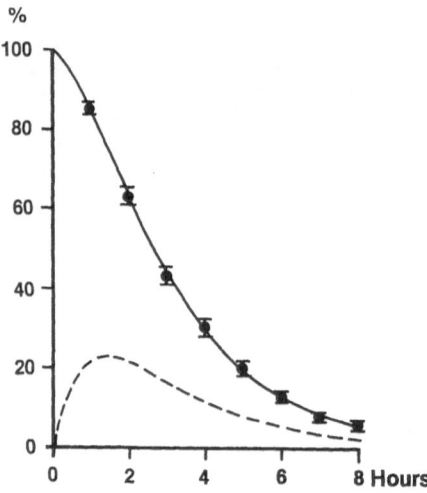

Fig. 12. Absorption of Actrapid MC. *Solid line* disappearance of radioactivity after subcutaneous injection of 12 units ^{125}I-labelled Actrapid MC 40 IU/ml into the femoral region of 33 diabetics (mean $\pm$ SEM) measured as described by Binder (1969). *Broken line* rate of absorption in percent obtained by derivation of the disappearance curve. (After Schlichtkrull 1977 b)

to stabilize the insulin (Sahyun et al. 1939), most likely because of an inactivating influence on contaminating enzymes. Lens (1947) was not able to confirm this stabilizing effect of zinc, possibly because the insulin examined was devoid of enzymes.

The absorption course of Actrapid after subcutaneous injection into the femur is shown in Fig. 12. The rate curve obtained by differentiation shows that it takes almost two hours for the insulin to be absorbed at maximum rate, viz. approximately 25% of the dose per hour. (Binder et al. 1967, Schlichtkrull 1977 b).

Comparing two neutral regular insulins of different formulation (Actrapid with sodium chloride, methylparaben and Leo Regular with glycerol, *m*-cresol) Berger et al. (1982) found that the absorption kinetics were virtually identical.

IV. Protracted Preparations

1. Introduction

Shortly after the introduction of the first acid insulin solutions the search for protracted insulin preparations started. The very first attempts to prolong the action of insulin included combination with gum arabic (1923), lecithin (1923), oil suspensions (1925), other proteins (1925) and cholesterol (1926); however, they were unsuccessful due to poor stability of the preparations, pain upon injection or too variable an absorption rate. Subsequently attempts were made to obtain prolonged effect by the combination of insulin with vasoconstrictory hormones, such as adrenaline and vasopressin, but these attempts were also abortive due to great variations in the clinical effect. Reference is made to Dörzbach and Müller (1971) for a review of the earliest attempts to prolong the action of insulin.

The first successful protracted insulin preparation was protamine insulin, introduced in 1936 by Hagedorn and co-workers. The principle was to depress the solubility of insulin at neutral pH using a basic compound. Protamines were,

Table 6. Formulation of protracted insulin preparations (1983)

Classification after timing of action	Preparations with examples of trade names	pH Acid	Neutral	Physical state d	a	c	Retarding principle	Species of Insulin p	b	p/b	h	Other
Short-acting	Insulin Zinc Suspension (amorphous), Semilente, Semitard		×		×		Zinc	×	×	×		
Intermediate-acting	Insulin Zinc Suspension (mixed) Monotard, Monotard HM, Lente, Lentard, Hypurin Lente, Neulente, Optisulin Long		×		×	×	Zinc	×	×	×	×	des-Phe
	Isophane Insulin NPH, Protaphane, Isophane, Insulatard, Retard, Hypurin Isophane, Neuphane, Humulin I		×			×	Protamine	×	×	×	×	
	Surfen-insulins, Komb-insulin, Depot-insulin	×		×			Surfen	×	×			
	Long-insulin		×		×		Surfen	×				
	Globin Zinc Insulin, HG-insulin, Globin	×		×			Globin	×	×			
	Protamine Zinc Insulins, (amorphous)		×		×		Protamine+Zinc	×		×		
Long-acting	Insulin Zinc Suspension (crystalline), Ultralente, Ultratard		×			×	Zinc	×	×			
	Protamine Zinc Insulins, Hipurin PZ		×		×	×	Protamine+Zinc	×	×	×		
Biphasic	Biphasic Insulin Rapitard, Biphasic		×	×		×	Zinc	×		×		
	Biphasic Protamine Insulins Mixtard, Initard		×	×		×	Protamine	×				

Abbreviations: d=dissolved, a=amorphous, c=crystalline, p=porcine, b=bovine, h=human

among other basic peptides (histones, globins, etc.), found to show the most pro-
mising effect. Since the first neutral protamine insulin suspension was not stable,
it was necessary to dispense this new preparation in two separate vials, one containing a phosphate buffer and the other an acid solution of protamine and insulin (showing the same timing of action as soluble rapid acting insulins when injected separately). The patient would then prepare sufficient suspension for a few
days by injecting buffer into the vial with the acid solution of protamine and
insulin.

    Later more stable protracted preparations were developed, still including the
combination of insulin with foreign proteins. It was not until the introduction of
the Lente preparations (Hallas-Møller et al. 1951) that protracted insulin preparations without added foreign proteins or synthetic compounds were obtained.

    The composition of commercially available protracted insulin preparations is
given in Table 6.

2. Protamine Insulins

a) Protamine

Protamine is the generic name of a group of strongly basic proteins present in the
sperm cell nuclei in saltlike combination with nucleic acids. Commercially available protamines are made from fish sperm and usually obtained as the sulphate
salt.

    Since protamines emanating from different families, genera and species of fish
vary as to peptide composition, it is desirable to specify the family, genus and species of the fish from which the protamine is isolated. Protamines used together
with insulin are normally obtained from salmon (salmine) or trout (iridine).

    Salmine and iridine are inhomogeneous and have been separated into two and
three main fractions, respectively (Ando and Watanabe 1969). Each of these fractions is probably also heterogeneous as shown for iridine (Ling et al. 1971), but
the different peptides having about 30 amino acid residues are very similar in
structure. The average molecular weight of protamine has been found to be approx. 4,300 for iridine and 4,250 for one of the fractions of salmine (Ando and
Watanabe 1969).

    Basic residues constitute about two thirds of all the amino acid residues in
protamines resulting in an isoelectric point of above 12. Salmine and iridine belong to the monoprotamines, which contain arginine as the only basic residue. In
addition these protamines contain relatively few other residues predominantly
Ser, Pro, Val and Gly.

    Being devoid of aromatic amino acid residues, protamines have no UV-ab-
sorption in the region 260–360 nm, thus any absorption in this range denotes the
presence of potential impurities, e.g. DNA or histones, which contain aromatic
residues and are of higher molecular weight.

    Protamines were earlier considered non-immunogenic (Kern and Langner
1939, Jaques 1949) and the observed immunological reactions to protamine have
been attributed to contaminants (Caplan and Berkman 1976). Allergic reactions
due to the protamine content of NPH preparations have, however, been reported
(Shore et al. 1975, Sanchez et al. 1982) and Samuel concluded that protamines

can be immunogenic in man and their use for medical purposes may lead to formation of antibodies (Samuel 1977, Samuel et al. 1978). Recently Kurtz et al. (1983) found evidence that the protamine-insulin complex is itself immunogenic, as they showed a high prevalence of concomitant circulating antibodies against insulin and protamine in patients treated with protamine-containing insulin preparations.

Anaphylactic reactions to protamine sulphate have also been reported (Nordström et al. 1978, Moorthy et al. 1980, Knape et al. 1981, Vontz et al. 1982, Weiler et al. 1985), and the possibility of an allergic reaction to protamine must be considered in patients who are allergic to fish (Knape et al. 1981). Stewart et al. (1984) found a 50-fold increased risk of a severe adverse reaction to protamine if protamine is administered to diabetics receiving protamine-containing insulin preparations. The toxicity of protamine has recently been reviewed by Horrow (1985).

b) Protamine Zinc Insulin (PZI)

The first stable neutral suspension was developed by Scott and Fisher (1936), who discovered that a surplus of protamine and zinc salt in small quantities (2 µg zinc/IU) could stabilize the neutral protamine insulin. This protamine zinc insulin (PZI) has a much more prolonged effect, which may last for up to 72 h (Colwell, 1947). The dissolution of insulin before absorption is presumably due to degradation of the protamine by the fibrinolytic tissue enzymes (Hagedorn et al. 1936, Hagedorn 1946, Bang 1946, Brunfeldt and Poulsen 1953). The protaminase activity of serum is inhibited by zinc (Brunfeldt and Poulsen 1953), which may explain the different timing of PZI and NPH.

PZI made according to the United States or European Pharmacopoeias contains amorphous as well as crystalline protamine zinc insulin. Freshly prepared this PZI contains mainly amorphous precipitate which will gradually be transformed to crystalline particles upon storage, leading to a more protracted effect. Physically stable PZI preparations can be made either by avoiding the zinc binding phosphate buffer (resulting in intermediate-acting amorphous PZI) (Schlichtkrull 1958) or by crystallizing the protamine insulin (cf. NPH) before the surplus of protamine and zinc are added (resulting in long acting crystalline PZI).

c) NPH

A stable PZI modification, NPH (Neutral Protamine Hagedorn) also called "Isophane Insulin", was developed by Krayenbühl and Rosenberg (1946) at Nordisk Insulinlaboratorium. They found that insulin and protamine brought together in isophane proportions (the condition in which neither insulin nor protamine is found in excess) at neutral pH, in the presence of a small amount of zinc and phenol and/or phenol derivatives (cresols) will form an amorphous precipitate, which is gradually transformed into tetragonal oblong crystals limited at the ends by pyramidal faces (Fig. 9 d). At pH 7.3 insulin and salmine co-precipitate in a 5:1 molar ratio corresponding to about 0.13 mg protamine per mg insulin (Simkin et al. 1970).

The following conditions are necessary for rapid and complete crystallization of protamine insulin: the protamine, insulin and auxiliary substances must be reasonably pure and the proportion between protamine and insulin nearly isophane. The isophane ratio varies with different protamine and insulin qualities and species as well as with pH, temperature, content of zinc and auxiliary substances. Zinc in a concentration of approx. 0.2 µg/IU is necessary for the preparation of the tetragonal crystals as is the presence of phenol or phenol derivatives. m-cresol is more suitable for the crystallization than the corresponding o- or p-derivatives (Krayenbühl and Rosenberg 1946) or phenol (Fullerton and Low 1970).

Insulin-salmine crystals contain insulin and protamine combined in a complex in a molar ratio of 8.5 to 1 (Fullerton and Low 1970). It is assumed that protamine is to be found in the interstices between hexamers but not as an ordered component of the crystal lattice (Simkin et al. 1970, Hodgkin 1974).

Zinc is present in the same amount as in rhombohedral crystals (cf. C.II.4) (2 atoms of zinc per hexamer) together with about 0.5×10^{-3} mol phenol (or phenol derivatives) per gram of protamine insulin corresponding to 22 mols of phenol per hexamer (Krayenbühl and Rosenberg 1946). Suspensions of such crystals are stable in the absence of protamine-degrading proteolytic enzymes, such as pancreatic enzymes, which may be present in impure insulin.

Graham and Pomeroy (1984) found marked differences in duration of action between different brands of NPH largely due to variations in crystal size and shape rather than to differences in insulin species.

3. Insulin Zinc Suspensions (Lente Insulins)

The Lente insulins were developed in the NOVO laboratories by Hallas-Møller and co-workers (1951, Hallas-Møller 1956), who elucidated the influence of zinc ions on the timing of insulin preparations. They showed that insulin preparations with protracted effect could be obtained by addition of small amounts of zinc ions provided that the preparations had a neutral pH and that no interfering (zinc binding) ions, like phosphate or citrate, were present.

Furthermore they showed that the degree of protraction at the same zinc concentration depended on the physical state of the suspended insulin particles, amorphous insulin particles having a shorter time of action than crystalline insulin particles.

This led to the introduction of three new protracted insulin preparations all containing approx. 80 µg zinc/ml (40 IU/ml): Semilente containing only amorphous insulin particles, Ultralente containing only crystalline insulin particles and Lente containing a 3:7 mixture of amorphous and crystalline insulin particles. Bovine insulin was originally chosen for the crystalline part and porcine insulin for the amorphous part. Later Monotard, having a composition like Lente with the exception that Monotard contains porcine or human insulin only, and Lente preparations, containing only insulin of bovine origin, have been introduced.

Preparations containing insulin derivatives (des-Phe^{B1} insulin, cf. C.XII) in the amorphous part have been investigated clinically (Bottermann et al. 1980).

The Lente insulins were originally developed in the search for preparations able to cover diabetics' insulin requirement with one daily injection. Adjustments may be made by mixing the three types of Lente preparations in different ratios.

In modern clinical treatment individual mixtures of intermediate-acting and rapid-acting preparations are often given more than twice daily. A regime where the basal insulin requirement is covered by Ultratard, while Actrapid is used to cover meals, has been described by Phillips et al. (1979) and Ward et al. (1981).

In the Lente preparations a certain proportion of the total amount of zinc is present as zinc ions bound within the suspended insulin particles, whereas the rest is present as free zinc ions in solution.

Schlichtkrull (1958) established an empirical relationship between the amount of bound zinc ions (in number of zinc atoms per insulin hexamer), the concentration of free zinc ions and the concentration of hydrogen ions (constant temperature, pH around 7.3):

$$Zn_{bound}^{4.0} = k \frac{[Zn^{2+}]}{[H^+]}.$$

At the constant pH value of the preparations this means that at constant free zinc concentration, the amount of bound zinc in mg/100 IU of insulin (proportional to the number of zinc atoms per insulin hexamer) will be constant independent of total insulin concentration.

A concentration of free zinc of approx. 0.05 mg/ml at pH 7.4 was chosen for the original Lente series. This leads to an amount of bound zinc of approx. 0.09 mg/100 IU of insulin.

A calculation of bound and total zinc based on a concentration of free zinc of 0.05 mg/ml is shown in Table 7 for three different insulin strengths; as seen the total zinc content relative to insulin (in mg/100 IU) is adapted to the various strengths in order to maintain constancy of the chemical composition of the solid phase and of the suspension medium, aiming at an unchanged protracted effect.

The composition of Lente preparations with respect to other auxiliary substances (cf. Table 8) is described in section C.V, but it should be emphasized that, for example, phenol is unacceptable as preservative, since its presence leads to a change of the physical state of the insulin particles and thus probably a change of the dissolution and timing properties.

In the manufacture of Ultralente or the crystalline part of Lente and Monotard, the insulin is dissolved in acid, sterilized by filtration and thereafter crystallized as described in C.II.4. After the crystallization, pH is adjusted to 7.4 and the correct concentrations of insulin, zinc and other auxiliary substances are estab-

Table 7. Calculated values of bound, free and total zinc content in Lente preparations containing 40, 80 and 100 IU/ml with the presupposition that the content of free zinc is constant

Insulin strength IU/ml	$[Zn^{2+}]$ free mg/ml	$[Zn^{2+}]$ bound		$[Zn^{2+}]$ total	
		mg/100 IU	mg/ml	mg/ml	mg/100 IU
40	0.05	0.09	0.036	0.086	0.22
80	0.05	0.09	0.072	0.122	0.15
100	0.05	0.09	0.090	0.140	0.14

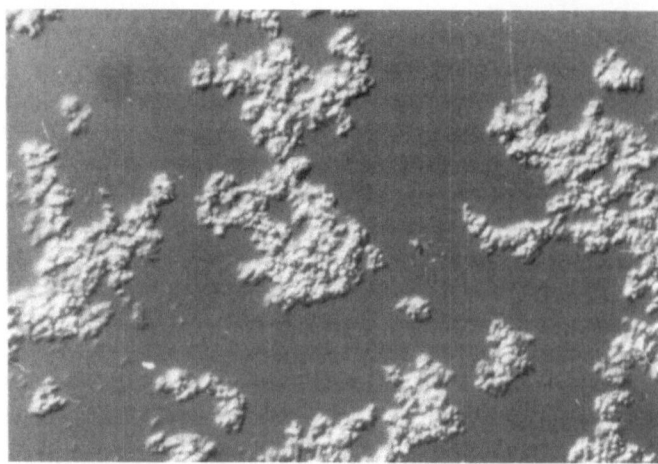

Fig. 13. Amorphous flocculation. Photomicrograph of Semilente showing loose aggregates of individual amorphous particles. 176 × magnification, using differential interference contrast technique

lished. The crystals formed during the crystallization are of the 4 Zn-insulin structure (cf. C.II.4) but X-ray studies have shown that complete conversion into the 2 Zn-insulin structure takes place during dilution and pH adjustment of the crystal suspension (Dodson, personal communication).

In order to obtain a constant and narrow size distribution of the insulin crystals a special seeding technique must be used (Schlichtkrull 1957b). This is advantageous because the timing of the preparations is to some degree dependent on the size of the crystals (cf. C.II.6, Fig. 11).

In the manufacture of Semilente or the amorphous part of the Lente preparations, the insulin is dissolved at acid pH and after sterile filtration the correct pH and zinc concentration are established. This leads to a precipitation of insulin as amorphous particles.

The size of the individual amorphous particles is about 1 μm. Microscopically, the amorphous particles are seen to form loose aggregates (Fig. 13). This flocculation is of importance for the physical stability of the preparations. Formation of lumps or flakes due to inappropriate storage has been shown to decrease with increased flocculation (Langkjær, unpubl.). Similar results have been reported by Haines and Martin (1961) for other suspensions.

The original Lente preparations were prepared using zinc chloride as the source of zinc ions but, as the amount of zinc ions present is the important factor, other zinc salts (e.g. acetate) may also be used.

For a detailed survey of the physical chemistry of the Lente insulins reference is made to Schlichtkrull et al. (1975a).

4. Biphasic Preparations

When using intermediate-acting insulin preparations the initial insulin effect is often too slight. A stronger initial effect can be obtained by mixing rapid- or short-acting preparations with intermediate-acting preparations (cf. C.VIII). The need for a stronger initial effect led to the search for stable mixtures of rapid-acting (dissolved) and intermediate- to long-acting insulin resulting in the development of Rapitard (Biphasic Insulin Injection) (Schlichtkrull 1959, Schlichtkrull et al. 1965).

Rapitard contains 75% crystalline bovine insulin suspended in a solution of 25% of mainly porcine insulin. The rationale for this preparation is the utilization of the difference in solubility between porcine and bovine insulin at specific values of pH and zinc concentration (cf. C.II.1). Due to the low solubility of the bovine insulin, only a small amount of the dissolved insulin is bovine.

The insulin crystals are prepared in the same way as the Ultralente and the crystalline part of the Lente preparation (cf. C.II.4 and C.IV.3). Crystallization in the presence of 7% sodium chloride leads to crystals containing 4 zinc atoms per insulin hexamer. After crystallization the preparation is diluted at constant pH (5.5) to the final concentration of insulin and auxiliary substances (i.e. 0.7% w/v of sodium chloride).

This leads to a crystal transformation from crystals containing 4 zinc atoms per insulin hexamer to crystals containing 2 zinc atoms per hexamer. The crystal suspension is later adjusted to pH 7 and mixed in the correct proportion with the separately prepared neutral solution of insulin. Rapitard is physically stable, the proportion of insulin in solution remaining constant during shelf life.

Two biphasic preparations have been introduced based on Isophane Insulin: Initard, a 1:1 combination of regular and NPH insulin, and Mixtard, prepared by adding 3 parts of regular insulin to 7 parts of NPH insulin. These mixtures are not physically stable, as some of the dissolved insulin is transferred to the solid phase. In Mixtard only about half the amount of the added regular insulin is recovered in solution (Galloway et al. 1982), whereas in Initard two thirds of the added regular insulin can be detected in the supernatant (Lykkeberg, unpubl.).

A biphasic insulin preparation utilizing the higher solubility of the insulin derivative, des-Phe^{B1}-insulin (cf. C.XII), as compared to that of the parental insulin has been introduced (Optisulin Depot) (Zoltobrocki et al. 1980).

5. Other Types of Protracted Preparations

Surfen insulin preparations of intermediate and long duration of action have been widely used in Germany. The prolonged action of these preparations is based on formation of a slightly soluble complex between insulin and the synthetically produced substance, 1,3-bis (4-amino-2-methyl-6-quinolyl) urea (surfen) at neutral reaction (Lautenschläger et al. 1937, Umber et al. 1938). The intermediate acting Depot-Insulin with 4.2 µg surfen/IU is an acid solution from which the surfen insulin complex precipitates as amorphous particles after injection. Komb-Insulin is a mixture of one part acid Regular Insulin and two parts Depot-Insulin, which is a neutral suspension of crystalline and amorphous surfen insulin in the ratio 3:1.

Several cases of allergic reactions to surfen have been reported (Kulpe 1958, Forck et al. 1975, Goerz et al. 1981) and the incidence of these reactions has increased in recent years (Goerz et al. 1981).

Bovine and later also human globin, the protein part of haemoglobin with four polypeptide chains varying slightly in structure from species to species, have also been used as complexing agents. *Globin insulin,* developed by Reiner et al. (1939) and dispensed in acid solution, is no longer widely used.

V. Auxiliary Substances

1. Introduction

The auxiliary substances used for the formulation of insulin preparations can be divided into five groups: 1. retarding substances (cf. C.IV), 2. preservatives, 3. isotonic agents, 4. buffering substances and 5. acid and basic substances for adjustment of pH.

A survey of auxiliary substances, other than retarding substances, used in commercially available protracted preparations is shown in Table 8.

2. Preservatives

As the individual dosage varies considerably from patient to patient multidose vials have to be used. Consequently, the preparations must be formulated with

Table 8. Auxiliary substances in protracted insulin preparations

Classification after timing of action	Preparation	Preservative	Isotonic agent	Other additives including buffering substances
Short-acting	Insulin Zinc Suspension amorphous	Methylparaben	Sodium chloride	Sodium acetate
Intermediate-acting	Insulin Zinc Suspension mixed	Methylparaben	Sodium chloride	Sodium acetate
	Isophane Insulin	Phenol and *m*-cresol	Glycerol	Sodium phosphate
	Surfen-insulin	Methylparaben	Glycerol[a] Sodium chloride[b]	– –
	Globin Zinc Insulin	Phenol, cresol or methylparaben	Glycerol	
	ZPI-Novo	Methylparaben	Glycerol	Sodium acetate
Long-acting	Insulin Zinc Suspension (crystalline)	Methylparaben	Sodium chloride	Sodium acetate
	Protamine Zinc Insulins	Phenol	Glycerol	Sodium phosphate
Biphasic	Biphasic Insulin	Methylparaben	Sodium chloride	Sodium acetate
	Biphasic Protamine Insulins	Phenol and *m*-cresol	Glycerol	Sodium phosphate

[a] acid forms = Depot, Komb.

[b] neutral form = Long

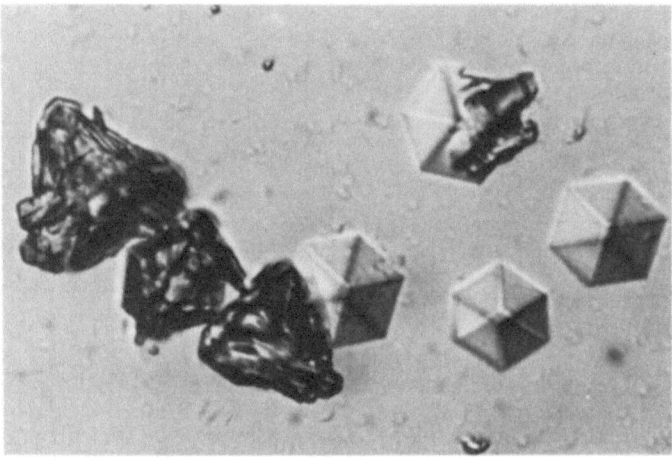

Fig. 14. Photomicrograph of Monotard modified by substitution of methylparaben with phenol, showing the appearance of abnormal crystals after storage for 6 months at 25 °C. (460 × magnification)

a suitable antimicrobial preservative. Selection of a proper antimicrobial agent is a compromise of efficacy, toxicity, compatibility with the insulin and interaction with the vial and the rubber closure (Allwood 1978). For instance, preservation of insulin zinc suspensions (Lente series) with phenol is not possible without influencing the physical stability of the preparation (Fig. 14), whereas methyl 4-hydroxy benzoate (methylparaben) does not exhibit this effect.

On the other hand, the presence of phenol (or a phenol derivative) is a prerequisite for obtaining protamine insulin crystals (NPH) (cf. C.IV.2.c).

The antimicrobial efficacy of phenols is generally considered to be better than that of the parabens (alkyl 4-hydroxybenzoates). Thus, Allwood (1982) compared the efficacy of various preservatives in different insulin injections and found neutral preparations with phenol or cresol relatively well preserved when compared to preparations containing methylparaben. Schade and Eaton (1982) inoculated 10 ml of neutral insulin solutions formulated with phenol with 5×10^5 bacteria commonly found on skin and found that the bacteria were killed within 24 hours. They also demonstrated a strong bactericidal effect of zinc ions at a concentration similar to that of the Lente series. Comparing the antimicrobial properties of different parabens O'Neill and Mead (1982) demonstrated that methylparaben in neutral solution is a potent preservative and superior to other parabens.

The concentration of the preservatives is affected by sorption (viz. adsorption and absorption) and in the case of parabens also hydrolysis. The distribution between water and a rubber closure was measured by Wallhäusser (1974), who found stronger sorption of phenol and m-cresol, especially, than of methylparaben. Rowles et al (1971) showed that phenol and m-cresol are not only absorbed by but also permeate the closure.

The hydrolysis of methylparaben was studied by Blaug and Grant (1974) who found that phosphate increases the rate of hydrolysis. The amount of methyl-

Table 9. Loss of methylparaben during storage of Lente when the preparation is in direct contact with the rubber closure (storage upside down). (Brange, unpublished)

	Storage at 4 °C		Storage at 25 °C
	1 year	3 years	1 year
Hydrolysis	2%	4%	9%
Sorption	7%	10%	12%

paraben disappearing due to absorption and hydrolysis during storage of Lente insulin is shown in Table 9.

The presence of the preservative has caused misinterpretations of the chromatograms obtained by analytical gel filtration of insulin preparations (cf. B.I.2).

3. Isotonic Agents

As with the preservative, the selection of a suitable isotonic agent is not a free option. Thus the use of sodium chloride is mandatory in the Lente series, because it is necessary during formation of the crystalline phase (cf. C.II.4 and C.IV.3). The choice of preservative and isotonic agent will affect the properties of the preparation, as revealed by the chemical stability (cf. C.IX.2) and the miscibility of neutral solutions with intermediate-acting preparations (cf. C.VIII.1).

The interaction when adding aprotinin to neutral insulin solutions has also been shown to vary with the formulation. Thus when glycerol is used as isotonic agent (low ion strength) a precipitation occurs which is not seen when using sodium chloride (Havelund, unpublished).

4. Buffering Substances

If the vial and rubber closure are of sufficiently good quality, proper pH is maintained without addition of buffer. Thus Jackson et al. (1972) found buffering of neutral insulin solutions unnecessary. In the Lente series acetate is used as buffer during crystallization at pH 5.5 and only negligible buffer capacity remains upon adjustment to neutral reaction. However, the preservative, methylparaben (pK$_a$ 8.4), possesses a certain buffer capacity (Tammilehto and Büchi 1968).

The presence of free zinc ions is prohibitive for the use of phosphate buffer in the Lente series due to the low solubility of zinc phosphate (Schlichtkrull 1958, Schlichtkrull et al. 1975 a). This also makes rapid-acting preparations containing phosphate buffer unsuitable for mixing with this type of preparation (cf. C.VIII.1).

VI. Characterization and Testing

1. Introduction

The different insulin preparations are subjected to a number of analytical tests in order to ensure their identity, and specified characteristics and uniformity. The various tests can be divided into groups after their application, one group covering the tests common to all the preparations and the other groups specific for certain special preparations. A historical review of the analytical control of insulin has been published by Stewart (1974).

2. Analytical Tests Applied to all Preparations

a) Control of Insulin Concentration

In the early days of insulin therapy biological standardization of insulin (cf. B.II.1) and insulin preparations was introduced as a necessary measure due to the large and varying content of impurities. Today this control is still based on biological standardization, even of the highly purified insulins, however, work is in progress to replace bioassay methods by analytical chemical methods (cf. B.II.2).

b) Control of Homogeneity of Insulin Suspensions

Control of the homogeneity of the filled vials is performed by nitrogen determinations on samples taken at regular intervals during the filling procedure. The results have to comply to specified limits.

c) Determination of pH, Zinc, Isotonic Agent, Preservative, and Species

The pH is of great importance for the physicochemical properties of insulin (cf. C.II), and it must be within narrow limits.

Like pH, the zinc concentration influences the physicochemical properties of insulin. The zinc concentration can be determined by atomic absorption spectroscopy as described in the British Pharmacopoeia.

The concentration of isotonic agent can be determined non-specifically by determining the freezing point depression of the solution/suspension or by specifically determining the concentration of the isotonic agent actually applied.

As the preservatives used in insulin preparations are strongly UV-absorbing, their concentration can be determined by UV-spectroscopy, if necessary after precipitating the insulin by addition of a surplus of zinc and adjustment of pH to a value where zinc is capable of precipitating the insulin.

Bovine insulin can be distinguished from porcine and human insulin by its ability to form so-called "stars" during crystallization under proper conditions (cf. C.II.4). A new, convenient and more sensitive method capable of separating bovine, porcine and human insulin is HPLC (cf. B.I.5).

3. Analytical Control Specific for Special Preparations

a) Protamine Insulins

Contamination of isophane insulin by proteases (potential contaminants from pancreas) can lead to digestion of protamine and a consequent release of insulin into solution. This phenomenon will lead to dramatic changes of the timing characteristics of the preparations and an analytical test for *protaminase activity* is therefore essential. The British and the European Pharmacopoeias describe a method of analysis for determining the proteolytic activity in Isophane Insulin by which the loss of weight of the isolated, washed and dried insulin protamine complex after incubation at 37 °C for 30 days is measured. Other more specific determinations of the sort of proteolytic activity have been described (Caygill and Ayling 1979), but the non-specific pharmacopoeia method has the advantage that it is a measure of the amount of insulin-protamine complex degraded. The determination of a rather small (relative) weight difference after isolating, washing and drying of the insulin protamine complex is inaccurate. The analysis may be improved considerably by determining the increase of nitrogen content in the supernatant.

It is of importance for the timing of action of the preparations that no insulin occurs in solution. The absence of *insulin in solution* can be determined by bioassay for all protamine insulins, or for Isophane Insulin by control of the isophane ratio as described in the following.

Deviations from the *isophane ratio* between insulin and protamine (cf. C.IV.2) can be controlled by isolating samples of the supernatant liquid and adding neutral solutions of protamine and insulin, respectively. If the supernatant liquid contains insulin the addition of protamine solution will cause the formation of turbidity; if the supernatant contains protamine the addition of insulin will cause the formation of turbidity.

b) Lente Insulins

As mentioned previously the total *zinc concentration* is of significance for all insulin preparations. For the Lente insulins it is, however, not only the total zinc concentration that is of interest but also the *distribution of zinc* between free zinc ions in solution and zinc bound to the suspended insulin particles (cf. C.IV.3). Therefore the zinc ion concentration in the supernatant liquid isolated after centrifugation is also determined.

The absence of *insulin in solution* may be controlled by bioassay but, as insulin is the sole protein present in the Lente insulins, the control can also be performed by non-specific determination of protein or nitrogen in the supernatant liquid.

For Lente and Ultralente preparations the *content of amorphous* insulin particles is determined (methods described in various pharmacopoeias). As the amorphous particles are soluble in a buffered acetone/water solution, the content of amorphous insulin present is determined as the proportion of nitrogen (equivalent to insulin) which can be extracted by this buffer. An alternative method of analysis has been described by Orr and Spence (1977). By this method the distribution of the differently sized amorphous and crystalline particles is determined using an electronic particle counter, whereby the proportion of amorphous particles can be estimated.

The *crystal size distribution* in Ultralente and the crystalline part of Lente, which is of importance for the timing of action of the preparations (cf. C.II.6), can be determined microscopically (Schlichtkrull 1957 a) or by using an electronic particle counter.

c) Biphasic Insulin Preparations

For the biphasic preparations the proportion of *insulin present in dissolved state* is of importance for the timing. This proportion is determined e.g. by nitrogen determination.

The *crystal size distribution* of Rapitard is determined as described above for Lente insulins.

4. Prolongation Tests

The timing of action of insulin preparations has been studied in rabbits, guinea pigs, mice, depancreatized dogs, healthy students and diabetics (both with stable and unstable blood sugar) using either strictly controlled conditions or conditions simulating daily life. Biological tests in animals are used for the control of constancy of the timing of action of an insulin preparation, e.g. from one batch to another, or during its shelf life until the date of expiry. Such tests for prolongation of insulin effect using either guinea pigs or rabbits are described in the pharmacopeias (British Pharmacopoeia 1980, Eur. Pharmacopoeia 1975, US Pharmacopoeia 1980). In these tests the prolongation of the hypoglycaemic effect produced by the prolonged acting insulin preparation is compared with the effect of the rapid-acting standard preparation. Figure 15 shows an example of such a test for prolongation of insulin effect where Insulin Monotard MC, fresh and stored, is compared with Insulin Actrapid MC. The test is performed according to the method described in BP (1980) using 36 rabbits in a cross-over design. The data recorded are the mean blood glucose values of the groups of rabbits obtained ½, 1, 2, 4, 6, and 7 hours after the injection expressed in percent of the initial blood glucose. Both Monotard preparations show prolonged effect compared to Insulin Actrapid MC, and analyses of variance followed by paired t-tests show no statistically significant (5 percent sign. level) differences between Monotard MC freshly prepared and that stored for 3 years at 4 °C.

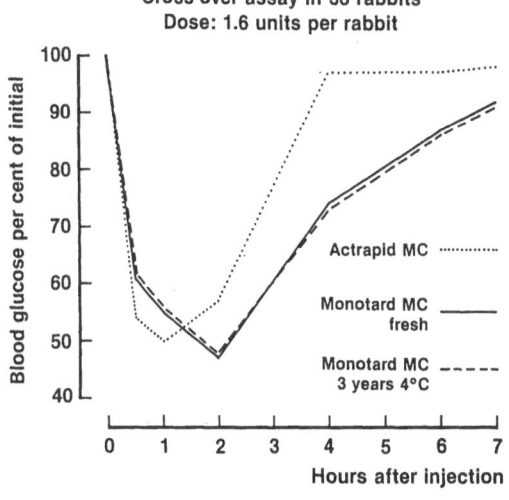

Fig. 15. Cross-over assay on 36 rabbits where the timing of action of Insulin Monotard MC after preparation and after 3 years' storage at 4 °C is compared with that of Insulin Actrapid MC. (Sørensen and Pingel, unpublished)

% of insulin eluted per 10 min

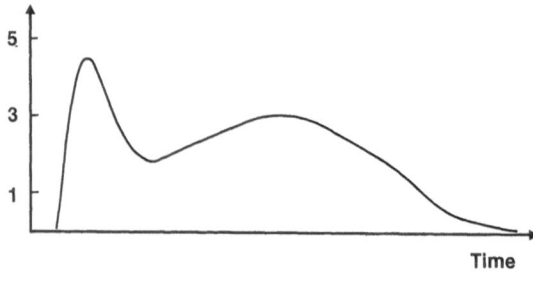

Fig. 16. In vitro elution profile of Monotard 80 IU/ml. Cell volume 10.0 ml. Eluent flow 0.19 ml/min. Temperature 37 °C. Time to maxima is dependent on the conditions of elution. In this experiment, approx. 1 and 4.5 h (Skelbæk-Pedersen, unpublished)

Time

An *in vitro absorption model* has been developed (Skelbæk-Pedersen, unpublished) to imitate the in vivo absorption of insulin preparations. The model consists of a "flow-through" cell with stirrer thermostated at 37 °C, and a filter fine enough to retain suspended insulin particles of different kinds. The cell is eluted with buffer, the composition of which imitates the composition of interstitial fluid. The eluate is collected in fractions in which the insulin concentration is determined. The result of such an experiment can be seen in Fig. 16, showing the elution profile of Monotard. The in vitro model allows a high degree of sensitivity and clearly differentiates the biphasic dissolution profile corresponding to the amorphous and crystalline insulin particles, respectively. An in vitro test based on similar principles, but without the same possibility to demonstrate biphasic action, has been published by Graham and Pomeroy (1984).

VII. Insulin Strengths

1. Introduction

The strength of insulin preparations is expressed in international units per ml or IU/ml. Since the discovery of insulin there have been a number of definitions of the unit of insulin. In 1923 it was decided to prepare a standard of Insulin with a defined specific activity. This led to the introduction in 1925 of the 1st International Standard of Insulin having a specific activity of 8 units per mg. This has been followed by the 2nd, 3rd and 4th International Standards of Insulin introduced in 1935, 1952 and 1958, the latter a mixture of bovine and porcine insulin and with a potency of 24 IU per mg. At present new international standards based on twice chromatographed species pure insulin (cf. B.II.1) are under way (WHO 1982).

The standardization of insulin samples relative to the international standards is described in section B.II.1. For a thorough survey of the development of the unit of insulin reference is made to the review by Lacey (1967).

2. Strengths of Insulin Preparations

The first insulin preparations contained only 1 unit per ml, but as the isolation and purification procedures became better, preparations of higher strength became available: 1922: up to 10 units/ml, 1923: 20 units/ml, 1924: 40 units/ml and in 1925: 80 units/ml (Scheller and Galloway 1975). For a long time preparations containing 40 and 80 units/ml were the two standard strengths produced. Because of reports of medication errors caused by the use of both U-40 and U-80 preparations (Watkins et al. 1967) the American Diabetes Association decided that only one concentration of insulin should be available in the United States. The concentration of 100 IU/ml was chosen by the American Diabetes Association, FDA and the insulin manufacturers in the USA and Canada, based on the following arguments: 1) the availability of syringes capable of accurately delivering small doses of concentrated insulin, 2) the trend toward adoption of the metric system in the United States and 3) the desirability of reducing the injection volumes. A trial with U-100 Lente and regular in children showed its safety and efficacy (Rosenbloom et al. 1971). Since then U-100 insulin preparations have been introduced in a number of countries, e.g. USA 1973, Canada 1975, Australia and New Zealand 1980, United Kingdom 1983, Denmark 1986 (in some cases paralleled by the withdrawal of all other strengths).

Arguments have been raised against the use of U-100 as the only strength. The main problem is the difficulty of accurately administering very small doses of high strength insulin, as in the case of children for whom dilution of the U-100 preparations is often necessary (Jackson et al. 1977). Cogswell and Simpson (1980) found that 24 out of 40 newly diagnosed patients required daily doses of 4 units or less some time during the first few years following diagnosis. The frequent necessity of diluting U-100 preparations makes for even greater confusion than with therapy based on the U-40 and U-80 preparations. The trend towards improving insulin therapy by dividing the daily insulin dose into two or more injections will also require smaller doses (Rosenbloom 1974).

If syringes with significant dead space are used for mixing different insulin preparations, greater problems arise with U-100 than with U-40 or U-80 preparations because larger insulin doses (up to 10 units) are contained in the dead-space (cf. C.X.3 and Table 18). These problems may to some degree be overcome by the use of properly designed insulin syringes with minimal dead space (Rosenbloom 1974).

Besides U-40, U-80 and U-100, other strengths like U-500 are available on special request and preparations containing up to 5,000 IU/ml have been described (Galloway et al. 1981 b).

Table 10. Insulin concentration expressed as mg of dry insulin (containing approx. 5% water) per ml and mmol/liter in preparations of different strengths

Insulin strength IU/ml	Insulin concentration	
	mg/ml	mmol/l
40	1.5	0.24
80	3.0	0.47
100	3.8	0.59

The influence of strength on the rate of absorption of the insulin has been examined by Binder (1969) and Galloway et al. (1975, 1981 b) who concordantly found that injection of high strength preparations leads to relatively lower absorption rates. If the variation in strength is small, like the change between U-40, U-80 and U-100, the changes in absorption rates will be insignificant (Galloway et al. 1975, Lauritzen et al. 1984). Lauritzen et al. suggested that the decreased insulin absorption rate observed with increasing concentration and increasing volume of the injected insulin solution (Binder 1969) is balanced when identical doses of U-40 and of the more concentrated, but less voluminous, U-100 are given.

Corresponding values for insulin concentrations expressed in different units are shown in Table 10.

VIII. Mixing Insulin

1. Insulin Mixtures

Many type I diabetics require a stronger initial effect in addition to the delayed action obtained with the intermediate-acting insulins. When mixing rapid-acting with intermediate- or long-acting preparations mutual compatibility must be taken into account (Table 11). Today, when neutral regular insulin is generally available, addition of the original acid regular insulin to the insulin zinc suspensions should be avoided as it results in pH shift, which may affect the time action of the insulin.

Phosphate-containing preparations (e.g. Velosulin and Hypurin) must not be mixed with preparations of the Lente-type, as the phosphate binds and precipitates the zinc ions whereby the insulin particles dissolve and the retarded action is lost (Langkjær, unpublished).

Table 11. Miscibility of insulin preparations

	Rapid-acting insulin	Intermediate- and long-acting insulin
Physically unstable mixtures, mixing is not recommended	Acid regular	Lente series[a] Rapitard, NPH, PZI
	Neutral regular	PZI
	Neutral regular (phosphate buffer)	Lente series[a] Rapitard
Physically unstable mixtures, mixing possible	Neutral regular (no buffer)	Lente series[a] NPH
	Neutral regular (phosphate buffer)	NPH
Stable mixtures that can be stored for at least 1 month	Actrapid (BP) Acid regular	Rapitard Globin, soluble surfen insulin

[a] Including Lente, Lentard, Monotard, Ultralente and Ultratard

Regular insulin when mixed with Protamine Zinc Insulin, with a great excess of free protamine in the latter, promptly precipitates the soluble insulin. The degree of precipitation depends on the physical state of the PZI; the amorphous type binds a greater part of admixed regular insulin than the crystalline type (Krayenbühl and Poulsen 1959).

Physically stable mixtures can be obtained by mixing Semilente, Lente and/or Ultralente in any ratio. Mixtures of Actrapid (BP-formulation) and Rapitard can be stored refrigerated for one month without affecting the individual timing characteristics.

The most commonly used insulin mixtures, regular/NPH and regular/Lente are not physically stable, as some of the soluble insulin binds to the protamine insulin crystals or precipitates with zinc, respectively. This is demonstrated in Tables 12 and 13. It appears that in both combinations some of the regular insulin precipitates immediately after mixing and the proportion of insulin remaining in solution decreases with time, with decreasing ratio between regular and modified insulin and, regarding regular/NPH combinations, with increasing strength of the preparations. Corresponding mixing experiments carried out with Actrapid of BP-formulation (methylparaben and sodium chloride) showed a higher degree of

Table 12. Percentage of added regular insulin remaining in solution after mixing Actrapid MC (USP formulation) with Isophane MC (NPH). The figures represent mean $\pm$ SD (n = 3). Insulin in solution was determined after centrifuging the mixtures. (Lykkeberg, unpublished)

Actrapid : NPH ratio	IU/ml	Time after mixing		
		5 min	1 day	30 days
1:1	40	78 $\pm$ 1%	73 $\pm$ 2%	66 $\pm$ 2%
3:7	40	49 $\pm$ 3%	47 $\pm$ 3%	44 $\pm$ 1%
	100	38 $\pm$ 5%	34 $\pm$ 2%	29 $\pm$ 3%

Table 13. Percentage of added regular insulin remaining in solution after mixing Actrapid MC (USP formulation) U-100 with a Lentetype preparation, Monotard MC U-100. The figures represent mean $\pm$ SD (n = 3). The mixtures were filtered and the insulin concentration of the filtrate determined using Bio-Rad protein assay (Bio-Rad Laboratories). (Langkjær, unpublished)

Actrapid : Monotard ratio	Time after mixing	
	2 min	10 min
1:1	93 $\pm$ 4%	85 $\pm$ 4%
1:2	71 $\pm$ 2%	61 $\pm$ 2%
1:3	47 $\pm$ 3%	36 $\pm$ 2%

precipitation in the regular/Lente combinations. Comparable results were reported by Nolte et al. (1983), who also found variation between different brands of insulin with respect to the amount of regular insulin remaining in solution after mixing with modified insulins. For this reason change of insulin brand should not be made without adequate adjustment of the mixing ratio.

The fact that some of the insulin precipitates does not mean that the quick-acting effect is lost, because a fast absorption rate will be preserved when the insulin is injected in freshly precipitated form. Thus, Berger et al. (1982) found no difference in serum IRI values in a comparison of separate and mixed injections of Actrapid and Monotard when injected immediately after mixing. A time-lag of 5 min between mixing and injection caused a somewhat delayed rise of serum insulin not observed when regular and NPH were mixed. Galloway et al. (1982) investigated the physical stability of NPH or Lente combinations with regular and found that the amount of insulin in solution decreased more rapidly in regular/NPH mixtures than in the corresponding regular/Lente combinations. The in vitro data correlated with clinical findings in a study, when normal fasting subjects were given the same mixtures. Based on these findings it was suggested that patients who use mixtures of regular with NPH or regular with Lente should be advised to administer their doses immediately after filling the syringe. In contrast to these findings Heine et al. (1984) reported that the onset of action is delayed when regular insulin is combined in the syringe with Lente insulin even when administered immediately after mixing. Mixing regular insulin with human Ultratard, Francis et al. (1985) found a blunting of the onset of action of the short-acting insulin and suggested compensating for this by increasing the proportion of short-acting insulin in the mixture (see also Table 13). Recently Colagiuri and Villalobos (1986) showed that the magnitude of loss of quick-acting effect in diabetics when mixing regular and Lente insulins depends on the time between mixing and injecting the insulin (see also Table 13), and Forlani et al. (1986), using glucose-clamp technique, found that the difference in insulin profiles in diabetics is not accompanied by a significant difference in glucose requirement and concluded that the slight delay in quick-acting effect when mixing Actrapid with Monotard seems clinically irrelevant.

When mixing two insulins in the syringe it is generally recommended to withdraw the rapid-acting insulin first. However, provided appreciable mutual contamination of the preparations during the withdrawal procedure is avoided, the mixing order is not significant. But it is important to follow the same mixing order, as a change often means that the actual mixing ratio will be changed too, dependent on the size of the dead-space of the syringe (cf. C.X.3 for further details).

2. Dilutions

When necessary, for instance, in the treatment of small children, insulin preparations may be diluted. The diluting medium should be of similar pH and composition as used in the preparation in question regarding preservative, isotonic agent, buffer and free zinc ions. Dilutions of insulin preparations with proper media can be stored at 4 °C for up to a month under adequate asepsis.

3. Addition to Intravenous Infusion Fluids

Addition of insulin to intravenous infusion fluids is used in the treatment of diabetic ketoacidosis, for insulin delivery during surgery in the diabetic patient, and for pregnant diabetics during labour. The infusion fluids to which insulin is most commonly added are glucose, sodium chloride, and sodium bicarbonate solutions.

In order to ensure that the insulin treatment is safe and effective a number of factors must be considered. As infusion fluids must be particle-free, only insulin preparations in which the insulin is in solution can be added. No precipitation or cloudiness should be present after the insulin has been mixed with the infusion fluid. Mixing must be thorough because an uneven distribution of insulin in the infusion fluid may expose the patient to a potentially dangerous, possibly lethal, dose of insulin (Bergman and Vellar 1982).

For safety reasons most hospital routines require that infusion fluids are used within 12 hours – or at the most 24 hours – after the container has been punctured. In this short span of time insulin is stable in most i.v. fluids. Other drugs added together with insulin may cause degradation of the insulin. Some corticosteroid and heparin preparations contain sulphite in amounts sufficient to destroy significant quantities of insulin. The stability of insulin in infusion fluids of esoteric or unknown composition cannot be predicted.

Adsorption of insulin to infusion equipment, probably as dimeric molecules (Browne et al. 1973), is the major source of insulin loss from infusion fluids. Although this problem has been treated in about 30 publications since 1951 no straightforward solution has been found and many contradictory results have been reported. Recent publications on this subject are those of Hoffmann and Rühl (1982), Mitrano and Newton (1982) and Hirsch et al. (1981). Insulin losses from 20% up to 80% have been found when 10–100 units of insulin is mixed with infusion fluids in 500 or 1,000 ml infusion containers.

Adsorption takes place within minutes and varies with the material, more insulin being adsorbed to hydrophobic than to hydrophilic materials (Sefton and Antonacci 1984). In the majority of the studies it was found that the percentage of insulin adsorbed decreases with increasing insulin concentration and that less insulin is lost when equipment with a smaller internal surface area is used. It has been reported that the addition of 0.1–1% of albumin to an infusion fluid will prevent the loss of insulin by adsorption (Hoffmann and Rühl 1982), or, at least, lower it to less than 20% (Schildt et al. 1978), and that adsorption of insulin can also be prevented by adding 0.5% of polygeline (Kraegen et al. 1975). The addition of the patient's own blood to insulin infusion fluid is effective in minimizing adsorption of insulin (Kerchner et al. 1980). Adding extra insulin to the infusion fluid in order to counteract the adsorption loss has been suggested (Schild et al. 1978); with this technique the error in insulin dosage will probably not exceed 10–20%. Recently Furberg et al. (1986), using a polyvinyl chloride infusion system, reported that optimal delivery of insulin in a mixture containing at least 100 IU of insulin in 500 ml of 0.9% sodium chloride can be achieved by filling the administration set with the insulin mixture, storing the filled system for 30 min, and flushing 100 ml of the mixture through the system before starting the infusion.

The loss of insulin by adsorption to the infusion equipment is of minor practical importance provided a standard procedure is strictly followed (Berger et al. 1981, Fort 1981), as the optimal insulin dosage is not known at the time the treatment is initiated and is adjusted periodically according to bedside glucose monitoring.

IX. Stability

1. Physical Stability

Stored as recommended the *rapid-acting insulin preparations* remain as clear, colourless solutions during their shelf life. The neutral solutions stand exposure to temperatures as high as 60–70 °C for up to an hour without physical changes. On the other hand, when the insulin is exposed to elevated temperature (above 30 °C) and concomitant movement, insulin fibril formation may take place resulting in precipitation of biologically inactive insulin (cf. C.XI). In acid regular insulin the fibrillation appears as an increase in viscosity, which Storvick and Henry (1968) observed after storage at 37 °C for 2 years. If insulin solutions are frozen the insulin will precipitate but will normally dissolve again when brought to ambient temperature after thawing.

The *prolonged-acting preparations* containing suspended insulin are reconstituted as homogenous suspensions upon shaking when stored correctly (2–8 °C). Insulin suspensions exposed to freezing usually change in appearance and become lumpy or granular due to aggregation of the insulin particles. The increase in particle size results in an increased sedimentation rate (Fig. 17). This has also been shown by Graham and Pomeroy (1978), who studied the effect of freezing on particle size distribution, sedimentation rate and bioactivity of different preparations. The crystalline insulin zinc suspensions showed the smallest changes, although some crystal damage was observed. No differences between frozen and unfrozen preparations were found in bioassay and prolongation tests. Havlová

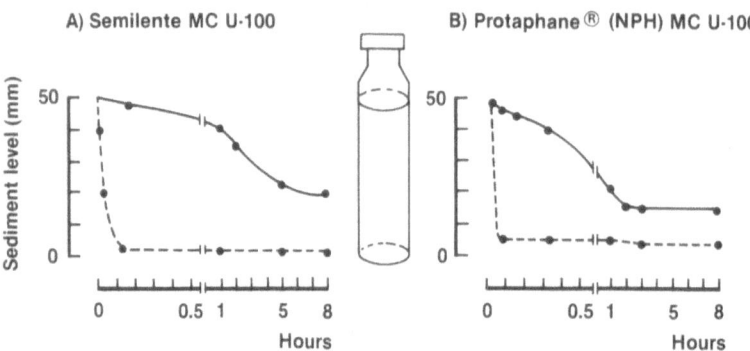

Fig. 17 A, B. Sedimentation rate of previously frozen (‐‐‐) and unfrozen (——) insulin suspensions. At time *0* the preparations are dispersed by turning upside down and left to settle. At different time intervals the distance between the upper level of insulin particles and the bottom is measured. Before exposure to freezing the insulin preparations were allowed to settle for 2 days

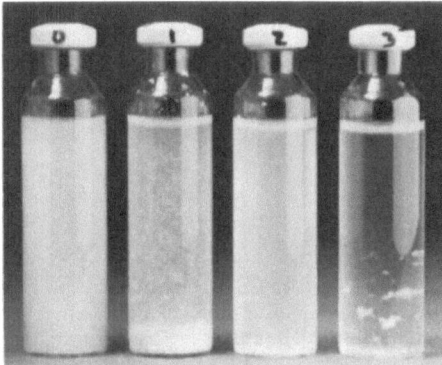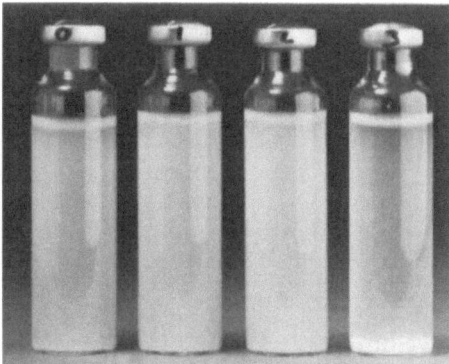

Fig. 18. Heat treatment of insulin suspensions. Vials of Protaphane (NPH) MC 40 IU/ml *(left)* and Lente MC 40 IU/ml *(right)* were exposed to the following temperature/time combinations in a water bath (from left to right): Untreated reference, 70 °C/24 h, 90 °C/2 min, 85 °C/30 min

et al. (1969), however, tested the effect of freezing on crystalline insulin zinc suspension and found that the frozen preparation was absorbed more rapidly than the unfrozen preparation. Therefore, it is not advisable to use insulin preparations which have been frozen, because it may be difficult to withdraw reproducible doses from lumpy and granular suspensions, and the timing may have changed as well.

Insulin suspensions stored at temperatures above 25 °C for extended periods of time may become difficult to homogenize. On exposure to temperatures above 50 °C the insulin tends to coagulate and form large lumps. Figure 18 shows the appearance of fresh and heat-treated Lente and NPH. The biphasic preparations containing soluble and crystalline insulin are also heat sensitive, as some of the crystalline material may dissolve upon heating and precipitate after cooling, possibly resulting in lump formation and deposits on the wall of the vial.

The physical appearance of insulin suspensions may also change if a drainage of liquid from sedimented insulin is allowed to take place. This may occur when vials in which the insulin particles have settled during a long period of storage are quickly turned upside down or revolved, leaving a part of the insulin isolated from the suspension. If these vials remain untouched for several weeks at room or higher temperatures the remaining liquid will gradually be drained from the deposited insulin resulting in lumps or flakes that are difficult to disintegrate upon shaking.

Slight changes in the colour of different preparations have been observed after long storage at 25 °C (Storvick and Henry 1968). In preparations containing phenol or cresol a yellow discoloration will occur after heat exposure possibly due to oxidation of the phenols.

A slight decrease of pH during storage of insulin preparations containing methylparaben is the result of hydrolysis of a small proportion of this substance into p-hydroxybenzoic acid (cf.C.V.2 and Table 9). Change of pH of Monotard during storage at different temperatures is illustrated in Fig. 19.

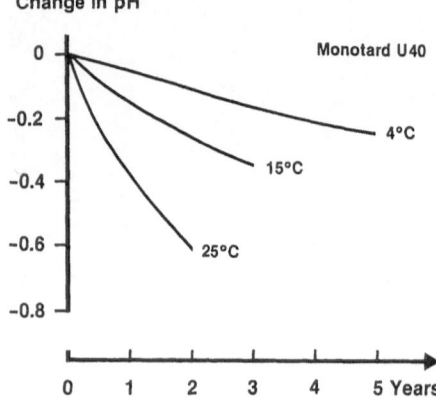

Fig. 19. Change in pH of Monotard MC 40 IU/ml during storage at different temperatures. The curves are based on results from a study including 8 batches

2. Chemical Stability

Like other proteins, insulin is not a stable entity but is liable to degradation by chemical reactions with molecules or ions in its vicinity, or to intra- and intermolecular transformations within the insulin molecules.

Whereas the stability of the pharmaceutical insulin preparations with respect to potency has been extensively studied, very little has appeared in the literature about the underlying chemical reactions leading to the loss in biological potency.

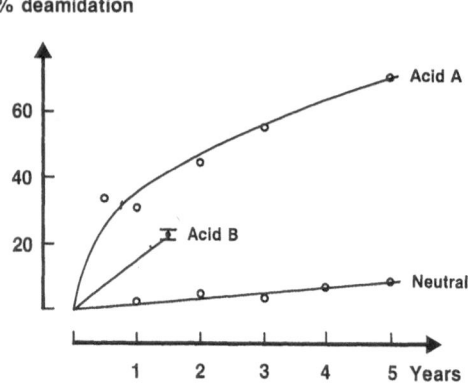

Fig. 20. Formation of deamidation products during storage at 4 °C of insulin solutions of different pH and composition. *Acid A* 0.1% methylparaben, 5% glucose, pH 3. *Acid B* 0.2% phenol, 1.6% glycerol, pH 3 *Neutral* 0.1% methylparaben, 0.7% sodium chloride, 0.1 M sodium acetate, pH 7. The desamido insulin content formed in *Neutral* and *Acid B* formulations was determined by basic disc electrophoresis followed by densitometric scanning of the amidoschwarz stained gels. Each point is the mean of analyses of 2–5 batches (*Acid B*±SD). (Brange and Langkjær, unpublished). The deamidation products formed in *Acid A* were determined by paper electrophoresis followed by staining, elution and spectrophotometric measurement of each component as described by Sundby (1962). Each point represents a single determination. (Pingel, unpublished)

Hydrolytic transformation of insulin in acid solution, with the liberation of ammonium ions and formation of deamidation products, has been reported by Sundby (1962), who demonstrated that monodesamido-(A21)-insulin is the prevailing derivative formed.

Jackson et al. (1972) compared acid and neutral solutions and showed that similar, but less pronounced deamidation can be observed in neutral regular insulin. Slow deamidation of insulin in neutral solution as well as in two different neutral suspensions was reported by Schlichtkrull et al. (1975a). A comparison of the deamidation during storage at 4 °C of two different formulations of acid solutions and a neutral solution is shown in Fig. 20.

At higher storage temperatures significant deamidation can also be observed in neutral solution (Fig. 21), in which the hydrolytic transformation has been shown to take place in the B-chain of insulin mainly at Asn^{B3} (Brange et al. 1983). The rate of deamidation in neutral insulin preparations varies with the formulation as shown in Fig. 22.

Formation of small amounts of covalent dimerization and polymerization products of insulin during storage of neutral preparations was reported by Schlichtkrull et al. (1975a). In neutral solutions this transformation varies with the formulation and the brand of insulin, as reported by Brange et al. (1982), the BP-formulation with sodium chloride and methylparaben being more stable than the USP-formulation with glycerol and phenol (or cresol). The reverse applies to

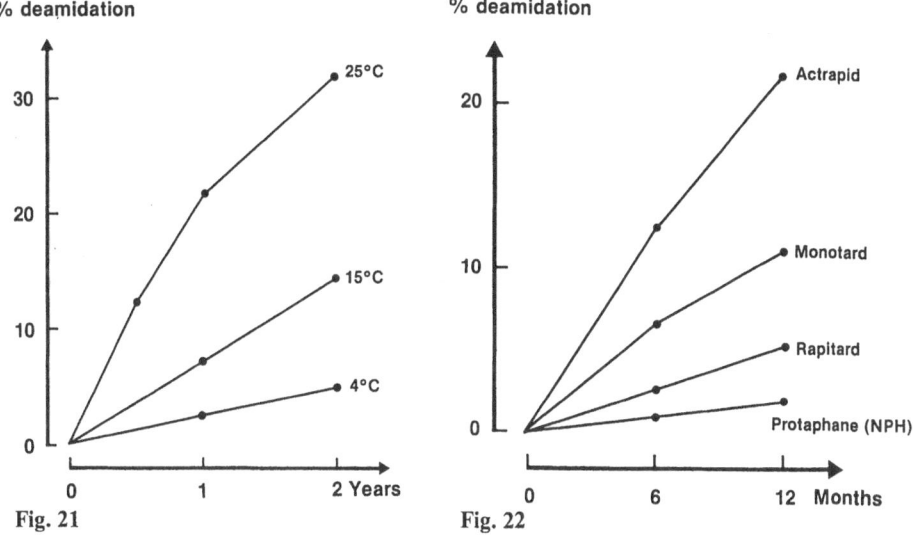

Fig. 21

Fig. 22

Fig. 21. Deamidation of insulin during storage of Actrapid MC (BP-formulation) at different temperatures. Each point represents the mean of analyses of 4–6 different batches. The desamido insulin content was determined by basic disc electrophoresis followed by densitometric scanning of the amidoschwarz stained gels. (Brange et al. 1983)

Fig. 22. Formation of deamidation products during storage at 25 °C of different MC insulin preparations. Each point represents the mean of analyses of 2–11 different batches. The desamido insulin content was determined by basic disc electrophoresis followed by densitometric scanning of the amidoschwarz stained gels. (Brange et al. 1985)

Table 14. Influence of formulation on the chemical transformation of insulin in neutral solution during storage at 25 °C for 6 months (Brange et al. 1982, 1983). For analytical methods cf. legends to Fig. 21 and Table 15

Formulation	% Deamidation		% Dimerization	
	Mean	SD	Mean	SD
Neutral regular USP (phenol or *m*-cresol, glycerol)	6.7	2.6 (n=5)	0.68	0.11 (n=4)
Neutral regular BP (methylparaben, sodium chloride)	12.4	0.9 (n=4)	0.34	0.13 (n=11)

the rate of deamidation (Table 14). The chemical stability of five different neutral formulations with regard to the formation of higher molecular weight products is shown in Table 15, from which is seen that variations in the formation of high molecular weight transformation products can also be observed within different formulations of protracted preparations.

The dimerization is mainly due to a reaction between an N-terminal amino group in one insulin molecule with a carboxamide group of a glutamine or an asparagine residue in the A-chain of another insulin molecule (Brange, unpublished). It is interesting that this dimer formation is of the same order of magnitude in the neutral solution (Actrapid) as in the insulin zinc suspensions (Monotard and Ultralente) (cf. Table 15). Apparently the intermolecular transformation proceeds within the hexamer, which is the common unit in the solution and in the crystals. This is supported by the fact that the rate of dimerization in neutral solution is independent of the concentration of insulin (Brange et al. 1983). Covalent insulin dimers, probably formed during production of crude insulin, and contained in the b-component (cf. A.IV, B.I.2), have been isolated from bovine b-component and extensively characterized by Helbig (1976).

The rate of transformation in protamine-containing preparations is higher, the difference being most pronounced at lower temperatures (Table 15). This is

Table 15. Formation (in percent) of high molecular weight transformation products of insulin in different preparations during 2 years of storage (Brange et al. 1984). The results are the mean of analyses by gel filtration on Biogel P 30 in 1 M acetic acid on 3–12 batches of each type of preparation

Type of preparation	Species of insulin	Temperature of storage		
		4 °C	15 °C	25 °C
Actrapid (BP)	Pork	0.11	0.46	1.6
Monotard	Pork	0.16	0.41	2.3
Isophane (NPH)	Pork	1.10	3.7	8.8
Ultralente	Beef	0.15	0.50	2.6
Zinc Protamine	Pork	1.6	5.5	15.5

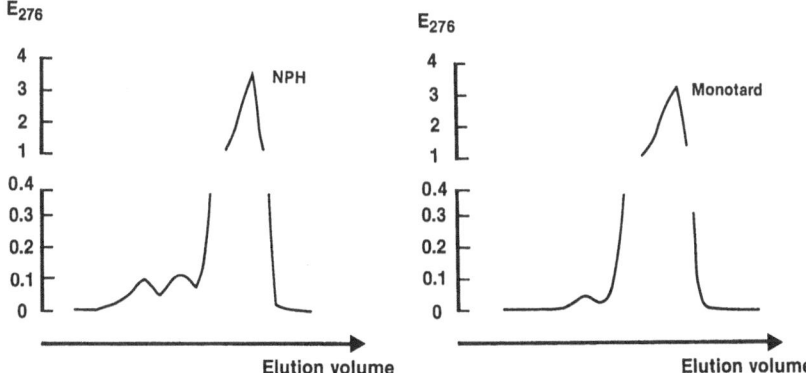

Fig. 23. Gel filtration of porcine Isophane (*NPH*) MC and *Monotard* on Biogel P 30 in 1 *M* acetic acid showing the appearance of an extra transformation product in NPH after storage of the preparations at 25 °C for 6 and 12 months, respectively (Brange et al. 1984)

partly explained by an additional formation of a chemical link between protamine and insulin. This covalent compound is easily demonstrated in isophane insulin stored for some time as a peak eluting before the covalent insulin dimer in analytical gel filtration (Fig. 23).

Formation of di-and polymerization products increases dramatically with increasing temperature, as shown for Monotard in Fig. 24.

Covalent dimerization products of insulin have been shown to circulate in diabetic patients treated with insulin (Robbins et al. 1985). These products have been demonstrated to originate from the insulin preparation by Maislos et al. (1986), who found that they accumulate in serum and constitute 28% of the mean fasting plasma immunoreactive insulin, probably due to slower metabolic clearance relative to insulin.

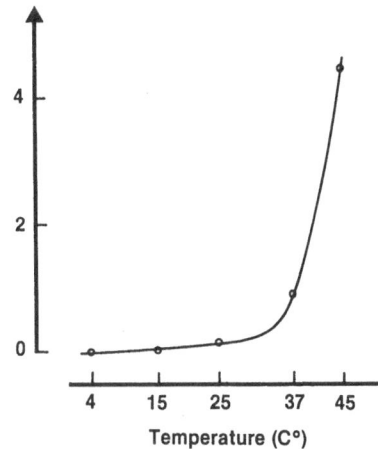

Fig. 24. Formation of covalent di- and polymerization products of insulin during storage of Monotard for 1 month at different temperatures. Each point is calculated on the basis of a study including four different batches. (Brange, unpublished)

3. Biological Stability

The biological potency of insulin is reduced during storage according to a first-order reaction

$$P(t) = P_o e^{-kt}, \tag{1}$$

where k follows the Arrhenius equation

$$k = e^{(\alpha - \beta/T)} \tag{2}$$

P_o is the original potency, P the potency after t months of storage at temperature T ($^\circ$K), and α and β are characteristic constants for the various insulin preparations. These constants for insulin preparations manufactured from recrystallized porcine and bovine insulins have been determined from accumulated stability

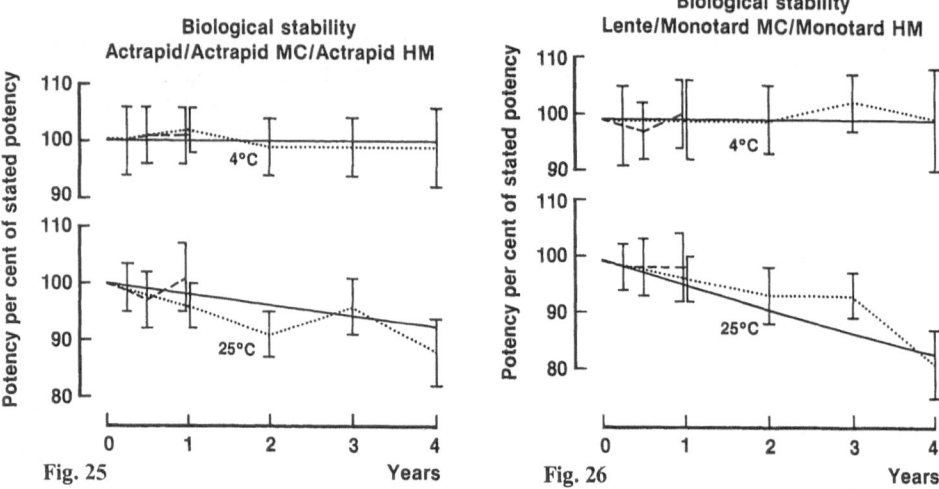

Fig. 25. Biological potency expressed in percent of stated potency after storage for different periods at 4 $^\circ$C or 25 $^\circ$C of Insulin Actrapid prepared from recrystallized porcine insulin (*solid lines* Actrapid), monocomponent porcine insulin (*dotted lines* Actrapid MC) or monocomponent human insulin (*broken lines* Actrapid HM). The *solid lines* are estimated from accumulated stability data obtained by the mouse convulsion assay (Pingel and Vølund 1972), whereas points connected with *dotted* and *broken lines* are the mean biological potencies with 95 percent confidence limits obtained by the mouse convulsion assay on 3–12 (mean 8) batches of the monocomponent insulin preparations. (Pingel, Sørensen and Sørensen, unpublished)

Fig. 26. Biological potency expressed in percent of stated potency after storage for different periods at 4 $^\circ$C or 25 $^\circ$C of Insulin Lente/Monotard prepared from either recrystallized bovine and porcine insulin (*solid lines* Lente), monocomponent porcine insulin (*dotted lines* Monotard MC) or monocomponent human insulin (*broken lines* Actrapid HM). The *solid lines* are estimated from accumulated stability data obtained by the mouse convulsion assay (Pingel and Vølund 1972), whereas points connected with *dotted* and *broken lines* are the mean biological potencies with 95 percent confidence limits obtained by the mouse convulsion assay on 3–11 (mean 7) batches of the monocomponent insulin preparations. (Pingel, Sørensen and Sørensen, unpublished)

Table 16. Time of storage of insulin preparations at various temperatures until biological potency is reduced by 2 percent/ 5 percent, respectively

Insulin preparation	Storage temperature			
	4 °C	15 °C	25 °C	40 °C
	years	years	months	weeks
Actrapid	36/92	5/13	12/31	5/14
Semilente	45/115	4/11	7/18	2/5
Lente	36/91	3/9	5/14	1/4
Rapitard	22/55	3/8	7/17	3/7
Ultralente	19/48	2/5	4/10	1/3

data by Pingel and Vølund (1972). For each type of insulin preparation equation (1) and (2) were fitted to data of biological potency (mouse convulsion assay) which were determined after storage of the insulin at different temperatures (4 °C, 15 °C, 25 °C, 37 °C, and 45 °C) for different periods ranging from a few months to several years.

The biological stability of insulin preparations manufactured from monocomponent (MC) bovine, porcine or human insulins is not essentially different from that of insulin preparations manufactured from recrystallized porcine and bovine insulins, as illustrated in Figs. 25 and 26. Hence the equations for the biological stability of recrystallized insulin preparations can be used for MC insulin preparations as well. Table 16 shows how long insulin preparations can be stored at various temperatures before they lose 2 or 5 percent of their biological potency. The figures are calculated from equations (1) and (2) using the estimated values for α and β (Pingel and Vølund 1972). These figures show that insulin preparations have a remarkably high biological stability especially when they are stored at a low temperature. For instance, all the insulin preparations will lose less than or about 2 percent in biological potency after storage for 19 years at 4 °C, 2 years at 15 °C, 4 months at 25 °C or one week at 40 °C.

The biological potencies of insulin degradation and transformation products formed upon storage of different insulin preparations at elevated temperatures are shown in Table 17. The products formed by hydrolysis of insulin possess full or nearly full biological potency, independent of the species of insulin and site of deamidation. Similar results were reported by Carpenter (1966) and Chance (1972) for bovine and porcine monodesamido-(A21)-insulin, respectively. In contrast, Easter et al. (1978) reported only a relative potency of about 60% for bovine monodesamido-(A21)-insulin. The full potency of the derivative formed in neutral solution explains why Actrapid in spite of significant chemical degradation possesses eminent biological stability even at higher storage temperatures (Table 16). The di-and polymerization products as well as the protamine-insulin product exhibit very low potency. However, the impact on the biological stability of the preparations only becomes significant after storage at very high temperatures (Fig. 24).

Table 17. Biological potency of transformation products formed in different insulin preparations. (Brange, Sørensen and Sørensen, unpublished)

	Isolated from	Species of origin	Bioassay method	Potency[c] IU/mg (95% conf. lim.)	Potency relative to insulin
Monodesamido-(A-21)-insulin	Acid solution	Pork	MBG[a]+MCA[b]	24.4 (23.5–25.4)	92%
		Beef	MBG+MCA	22.5 (21.4–23.4)	85%
Monodesamido-(B-3)-insulin	Actrapid	Pork	MCA	25.9 (22.6–30.0)	97%
Covalent insulin dimer	Ultralente (porcine)	Pork	MBG	4.4[d] (3.5–5.4)	15%
Covalent insulin dimer	Semilente	Pork	MBG	3.8[d] (2.9–4.7)	13%
Covalent protamine insulin complex	Isophane (NPH)	Beef	MBG	1.2[d] (0.9–1.5)	4%
Insulin polymerization product (MW 30.000)	Semilente	Pork	MBG	0.4[e] (0.2–0.6)	<2%

[a] Mouse Blood Glucose Assay (modified BP method C)
[b] Mouse Convulsion Assay (BP method)
[c] Based on dry insulin-component containing 14.5% nitrogen
[d] Slight protracted effect
[e] Strong protracted effect, wherefore a PZI preparation was used as standard

When a vial of insulin is exposed to sunlight a hundredfold increased loss of biological activity has been observed, as compared to storage in the dark at the same ambient temperature for the same length of time (Sundby, unpublished).

4. Immunogenicity Studies

Monodesamido-(A21)-insulin, dimerization- and polymerization products have been tested in rabbit immunization experiments and found not to be significantly more immunogenic than the parent insulin (Schlichtkrull et al. 1975a). The low immunogenicity of monodesamido-(A21)-insulin has later been confirmed by Kasama et al. (1981).

Deamidation products isolated from Actrapid or Semilente and the covalent protamine insulin compound isolated from isophane (NPH)-insulin after accelerated storage have also been found to be of low immunogenicity in rabbits (Figs. 27 and 28).

X. Storage and Use of Insulin

1. Storage

To ensure optimal preservation of the quality (characteristics) during shelf-life insulin preparations should be stored in the dark between 2 and 8 °C, freezing

**Average binding
of 125I-insulin**

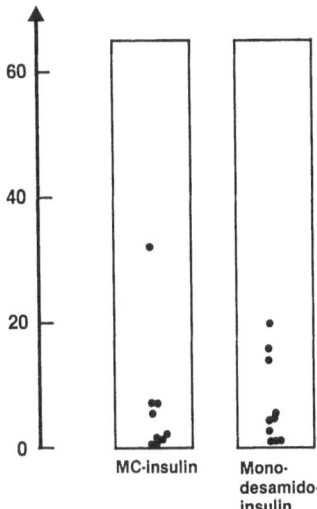

Fig. 27. Groups of 10 rabbits immunized twice weekly with neutral solutions of porcine MC insulin and porcine monodesamido insulin isolated from Actrapid MC stored at 37 °C for 3 months, 20 IU with Freund's incomplete adjuvant. Each dot represents the average binding of ^{125}I-insulin (cf. legend to Fig. 28) during the first 70 days of immunization of one rabbit. (Brange et al. 1983)

% bound 125I-insulin

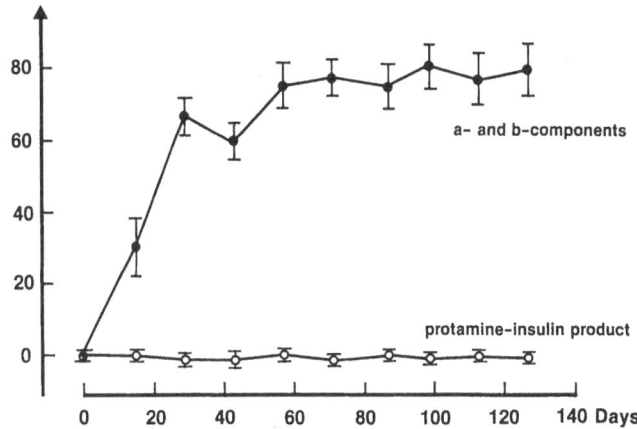

Fig. 28. Groups of 10 rabbits immunized twice weekly with a mixture (1:1) of acid solutions of porcine a- and b-component (cf. B.I.2) and high molecular transformation products, including 50% of covalent protamine-insulin product isolated by gel filtration from Isophane MC (NPH) after storage of the preparation for 3 months at 37 °C, 40 µg with Freund's incomplete adjuvant. The *ordinate* represents the antibody level as determined by the percent bound ^{125}I-beef insulin in serum diluted 1:3 (Schlichtkrull et al. 1972), the *abscissa* represents the time of sampling since the start of immunization. Each point represents the mean ±SEM, (Brange et al. 1984)

should be avoided. When necessary insulin can be stored for several weeks at temperatures not exceeding 25 °C without any significant change in biological activity. A vial in use can be stored at an ambient temperature not exceeding 25 °C to make the injection more comfortable.

Storage at higher temperatures should be avoided as it may alter the physical properties of the insulin preparations (cf. C.IX.1). Thus, precipitation may occur in regular insulin and the insulin suspensions may become granular in appearance or clumped in large particles resulting in loss of activity, changed timing characteristics or, at least, in difficulties in withdrawing the proper doses.

It is important to store insulin in the dark as exposure to direct sunlight and even diffuse daylight results in decreased biological activity (cf. C.IX.3).

Insulin preparations should not be allowed to freeze, as freezing induces particle aggregation, which makes it difficult to withdraw the correct dosage (cf. C.IX.1).

Sedimented insulin suspensions that have been stored for more than a few weeks should be homogenized prior to restorage, as their resuspendability may otherwise be affected (cf. C.IX.1).

2. Withdrawal of Insulin from the Vial

Before the withdrawal of insulin the vial should be inspected to ensure that the preparation has not changed in appearance. No discoloration must be observed, nor in solutions any precipitation found. The insulin suspensions are usually homogenized by gentle shaking, avoiding froth or bubbles which may make it difficult to measure the correct dose as insulin particles accumulate in the froth. If, however, the suspension is not completely dispersed it is necessary to shake the vial vigorously until complete homogenization. Then the vial should be allowed to stand until the froth has disappeared. Just before withdrawal the insulin should be homogenized again by turning the vial upside down several times. If the suspension has become granular or still contains lumps of insulin it should not be used.

The sterilized and separately packed disposable syringes and needles are most convenient to use. If reusable glass syringes are to be used, the proper sterilization procedure must be followed. The syringe should preferably be boiled in water for 5–15 min before each injection, alternatively, the syringe may be stored in 70% ethyl alcohol or 91% isopropyl alcohol (Purintun and McGrane 1972). In order to avoid dilution or contamination of the insulin before withdrawal, water or alcohol must be completely removed from the syringe by pushing the plunger up and down several times. For disinfection of the rubber closure ethyl alcohol (industrial methylated spirit) or isopropyl alcohol may be used. Surgical or medicated spirit which contains skin irritating additives must not be used; other disinfectants, e.g. solutions of benzalkonium chloride, cetrimonium bromide, chlorhexidine, etc. are not advisable, as even minimal contamination with these, induced by the needle perforating the rubber surface, can cause changes of the preparation, e.g. by precipitating soluble insulin.

Before withdrawal of the desired dose from the vial a corresponding volume of air is injected into the air space of the vial, taking care to avoid bubble formation.

After use glass syringes should be rinsed to remove traces of insulin which, when the syringe is boiled or immersed in alcohol, may coagulate and block the needle during the next injection. Clogging of the needle has been observed in rare cases, especially with U-100 suspensions. Usually this clogging can be prevented by correcting the sterilization procedure or by using disposable syringes. In order to prevent plugging during injection, the injection should be completed within 5 seconds after the skin has been penetrated by the needle (Galloway et al. 1976).

3. Mixing Techniques

When mixing two insulins in the syringe mutual contamination of the two vials should be avoided (cf. C.VIII.1). The size of the dead space in the conventional syringes varies from 0.05 to 0.1 ml and, as the first drawn insulin occupies the dead space volume, a change in the mixing order, model of syringe or insulin strength will also change the ratio between the two components. This is shown in Table 18. Arnott et al. (1982) compared mixing of Actrapid and Monotard in syringes with significant dead space and minimal dead space. They concluded that the latter type should be recommended for patients who inject mixed insulins, because the minimal dead space syringes are more accurate and the order of mixing is less relevant.

Mixtures of regular and retarded insulins normally have to be injected immediately after they have been drawn into the syringe in order to preserve their individual timing characteristics. Regarding compatibility between the different insulin preparations cf. C.VIII.1.

4. Preloading of Syringes

Insulin particles settle quite rapidly on standing. Therefore it is recommended to inject suspensions immediately after they have been drawn into the syringe. Some patients, however, are not able to withdraw the insulin by themselves and may therefore need to have their syringe preloaded. The preferred type of syringe for this purpose is the disposable syringe with minimal dead space, as this has been

Table 18. Effect of size of dead space, insulin strength and mixing order on actual doses delivered after mixing in the syringe. Intended dose: *10 U regular insulin* with *20 U protracted insulin*. The figures represent the actual doses in international units calculated under the assumption that the preparations are completely mixed in the syringe

Insulin drawn up first	0.06 ml dead space		0.10 ml dead space	
	U-40	U-100	U-40	U-100
Regular (R)	11.5 R	13.3 R	12.4 R	15.0 R
	18.5 P	16.7 P	17.6 P	15.0 P
Protracted (P)	9.3 R	8.3 R	8.8 R	7.5 R
	20.7 P	21.7 P	21.2 P	22.5 P

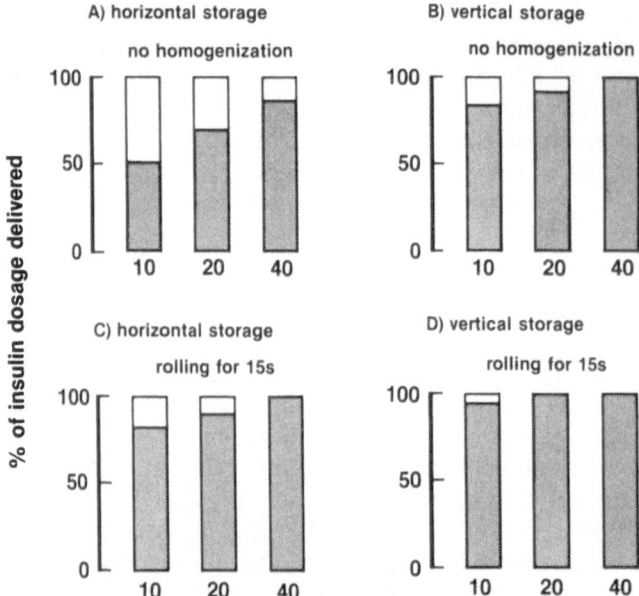

Fig. 29 A–D. Preloading three different doses (10, 20 and 40 IU) of ^{125}I-labelled Insulin Zinc Suspension (mixed) 40 IU/ml (Lente MC and Monotard MC) in disposable syringes (dead space 0.06 ml). After storing the syringes in horizontal (**A, C**) or vertical (**B, D**) position for 24 hours the insulin was expelled either without any previous homogenization (**A, B**) or immediately after rolling the syringe for 15 seconds between the palms of the hands (**C, D**). The percentage of the intended dosages actually delivered was determined by relating the radioactivity of the expelled volumes to the activity of corresponding accurately measured homogeneous suspensions. (Langkjær and Brange 1982)

shown to ensure correct dosage after having been preloaded for up to 3 days without taking special precautions (Langkjær and Brange 1982). If disposable syringes with significant dead space have to be used, a dose loss may occur due to sedimented insulin being retained in the dead space. As shown in Fig. 29, the relative loss varies with dose size and storage position, but the loss can be prevented by storing the syringe in a vertical position with the needle upwards and rolling the syringe between the palms of the hands for about 15 seconds to disperse the insulin particles prior to injection. The syringe should never be stored with the needle downwards allowing the particles to settle on top of the needle as this may cause plugging of the needle during injection.

From a sterility point of view preloading of syringes for a short period is no problem, provided adequate aseptic precautions are followed. Oberly et al. (1979), who tested the sterility of syringes preloaded with NPH, did not find any significant bacterial growth even after storage for up to 12 weeks.

XI. Insulin for Delivery Systems

1. Introduction

The subcutaneous injection of insulin does not provide optimal metabolic control, as this therapy is not able to mimic the delicate minute by minute modulation of insulin secretion which in normal persons occurs in relation to meals, exercise, etc. The prospects of decreasing the risk of late complications have, however, stimulated attempts to improve the therapy. Although good metabolic control with near normal glycemia has been demonstrated by using multiple (4–8) daily injections, the inconvenience of such a large number of injections precludes a widespread use of this regime.

In the past several years steadily increasing efforts have been directed towards developing sophisticated insulin delivery devices able to supply insulin continuously throughout 24 hours with alternating basal delivery and increments in relation to meals.

Development of such devices has taken two paths. *Closed-loop systems* regulate insulin delivery on the basis of continuously measured glucose concentration, but the lack of a stable portable glucose sensor has limited their use to hospitalized diabetics (Albisser et al. 1974, Pfeiffer et al. 1974). *Open-loop systems* (without glucose sensor) infuse insulin according to a preprogrammed schedule (Slama et al. 1974, Pickup et al. 1980).

Today only externally worn infusion systems (insulin pumps) are in widespread use, but prototypes of implantable insulin pumps have already been used in diabetics (Buchwald et al. 1981, Irsigler et al. 1981, Schade et al. 1982 a).

Insulin pumps are regarded as experimental instruments to be used in controlled research rather than a current therapeutic option (Marliss 1982, Lauritzen and Pramming 1984), and their use requires careful patient selection and available care by skilled professionals (American Diabetes Association 1985).

Recently a new portable insulin delivery system, the NovoPen, solving some of the problems of multiple daily injections, has become available. Having the size and appearance of a fountain pen it delivers a metered dose from a disposable cartridge by pressing a button without the need for handling vials, syringes etc. and it allows patients and, especially, diabetic children to inject themselves more conveniently, rapidly and with better dosage accuracy. Using the NovoPen, Jefferson et al. (1985) assessed a multiple injection regimen in diabetic adolescents and found that after a three month study period 8 out of 10 patients wished to continue with the regimen, finding that the advantages it offered outweighed the inconvenience of multiple injections. In another study 27 of 31 patients preferred NovoPen to a conventional twice daily regimen even though it necessitated four injections (Walters et al. 1985).

2. Use of Present Insulin Solutions in Infusion Pumps

Although neutral solutions of insulin can be stored for several years at room temperature without significant physical change (cf. C.IX) the use of insulin pumps has been complicated by the precipitation of insulin (Lougheed et al. 1980, Buchwald et al. 1980), especially when the pump design is based upon a peristaltic system (Irsigler and Kritz 1979, Jackman et al. 1980, Prestele et al. 1980, James et al. 1981, Schade et al. 1981).

Such precipitates, which may result in obstruction of the flow-system and especially of the catheter, can be due to the formation of amorphous particles of insulin (isoelectric precipitation), insulin crystals or insulin fibrils. The inconsistent terminology used when referring to these precipitates may have been a deterrent to solving many of the problems encountered when using insulin in pumps (Ege 1986).

The amorphous or crystalline precipitation is usually caused by zinc or various other divalent metal ions leaching from materials or by a lowering of the pH due to carbon dioxide diffusion or to leaching of acid substances from reservoir or tubing materials. (Melberg et al. 1987). This kind of precipitation can be prevented by selection of suitable materials for construction of the pump.

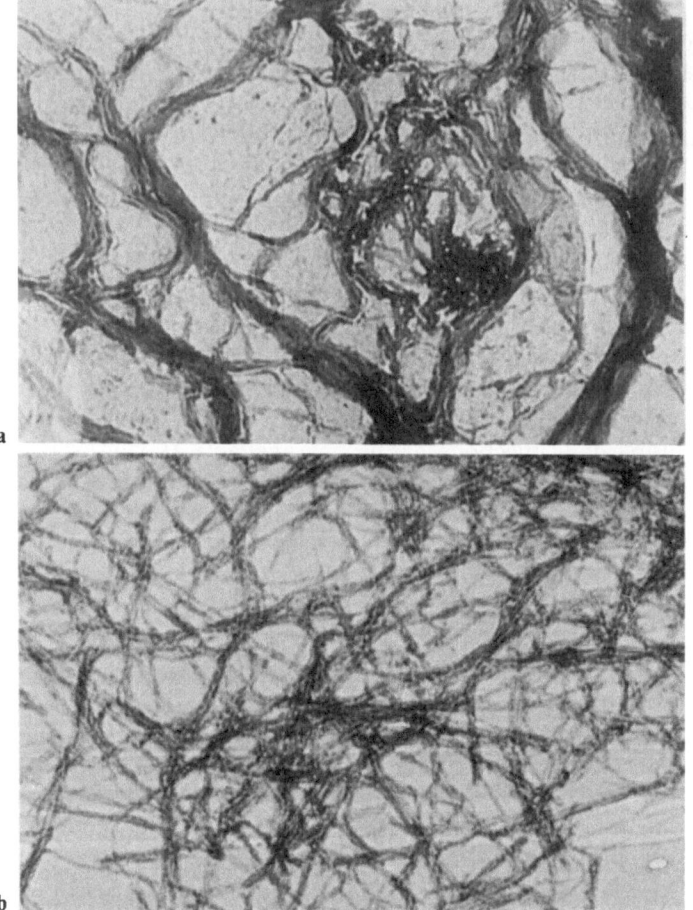

Fig. 30. Insulin fibrils × 100,000 formed at **a** 37 °C and **b** 80 °C. (Transmission electron microscopy)

The tendency of insulin to form insoluble fibrils under a variety of conditions by a non-covalent polymerization is more difficult to avoid. The promotion of insulin fibril formation by heat was first described by du Vigneaud et al. (1928) and Krogh and Hemmingsen (1928), and later extensively studied by Waugh (1946, 1948, 1954, 1957, Waugh et al. 1953). The interactions between molecules in insulin fibrils are mainly hydrophobic (Waugh et al. 1953) and seem to be of the parallel β-sheet type (Burke and Rougvie 1972). The formation of fibrils requires a monomerization of the insulin and a change in monomer conformation (Brange et al. 1987). Different forms of insulin fibrils are illustrated in Fig. 30. Fibril formation is also accelerated if insulin is exposed to hydrophobic surfaces (interfaces), which explains why different materials used in pumps influence the physical stability very differently (Brange et al. 1982, Lougheed et al. 1983, Feingold et al. 1984).

Schade et al. (1982 b) examined insulin fibrils by electron microscopy and concluded that the morphologic appearance of the insulin precipitated in vivo in the pump reservoir was not entirely reproduced by in vitro methods of insulin precipitation.

The requirements to the purity of insulin for continuous subcutaneous infusion can be expected to be very high if an immunological response, e.g., antibody formation or allergy, is to be avoided. The stimulation of the immune system is probably more intensive with an indwelling catheter supplying the insulin to a depot (pool) at the same infusion site for several days or weeks. Thus, Lauritzen et al. (1982) reported a surprisingly high antibody formation during subcutaneous infusion, and Pietri and Raskin (1981) found that allergic skin reactions, which occurred at the site of infusion with purified porcine insulin (Lilly) ceased on transfer to monocomponent insulin (Novo). Similar experience was reported by Levandoski et al. (1982), who obtained a dramatic reduction in nodule formation after changing from Iletin II to Actrapid. The physical stability of neutral insulin solutions with respect to fibrillation has been found to decrease with increasing purity of the insulin. This partly explains the difference in physical stability observed between different brands of highly purified neutral regular insulin, which were shown to differ considerably with respect to content of insulin dimers and polymers (Brange et al. 1982).

The contact with various polymer materials used in infusion pump systems impairs the chemical stability of insulin (Grau 1985, Melberg et al. 1987). The deterioration of the insulin is particularly profound when the material is gamma irradiated PVC (Melberg et al. 1987). Substances leached from the polymer material have been shown to be mainly responsible for the chemical transformation of insulin (Havelund, unpublished).

3. Physical Stabilization of Insulin Solutions

Much effort is being invested in the development of stable insulin formulations, particularly for implantable pumps. Evaluation of the physical stability at elevated temperatures of insulin solutions in ampoules and vials has been performed by rotation on a wheel (Thurow 1980) or by horizontal shaking of normal insulin vials placed in vertical positions (Brange and Havelund 1983 a).

   The requirements for introducing fibril-inhibitory additives include that the substance must be physiologically acceptable and compatible not only with the insulin and the auxiliary substances, but also with the pump materials. Furthermore it must be without negative influence on the insulin quality, viz. chemical stability, timing, immunogenicity, etc. Improvements in the physical stability of neutral insulin solutions have been reported by addition of autologous serum (Albisser et al. 1980), polypropylene glycol (Irsigler et al. 1981, Grau et al. 1982, Thurow and Geisen 1984), glycerol (Buchwald et al. 1981, Blackshear et al. 1983), carbohydrate (Brange and Havelund 1983b), different non-ionic and ionic surfactants containing a long aliphatic group (Lougheed et al. 1983) and calcium ions (Brange and Havelund 1983a). Bringer et al. (1981) prevented aggregation in acid solutions by addition of dicarboxylic amino acids, which, however, were without effect in neutral solution. Unfortunately, carbohydrates and glycerol have been found to impair the chemical and biological stability of the insulin (Brange et al. 1982, Brange and Havelund 1983b) and the use of synthetic detergents for long term infusion is questionable. The damaging effect of glycerol has been shown to be correlated with the purity of the glycerol, aldehyde impurities being responsible for the degradation of insulin (Havelund, unpublished). Sulphated insulin (cf. C.XII) having a biological potency of 20% of that of insulin has been found more resistant to fibrillation than other stabilized insulins (Albisser et al. 1982), possibly due to a high degree of heterogeneity (purity factor, cf. C.XI.2).
   Calcium ions, which probably play an important role for the storage of insulin in the pancreatic B-cell as well (Howell et al. 1978), are particularly effective in stabilizing higher concentrations of insulin (Fig. 31), and improve the physical stability without affecting the quality of the insulin. The positive effect of calcium ions is probably explained by binding of these ions to specific sites within the hexamer (Sudmeier et al. 1981), thereby protecting and stabilizing the hexameric structure.

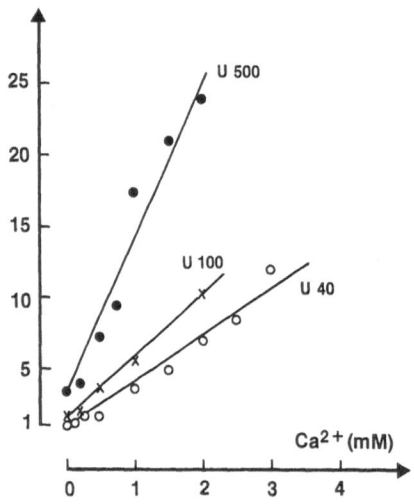

Fig. 31. The effect of calcium ions on the relative physical stability of neutral porcine insulin solutions (0.2% phenol, 1.6% glycerol) of different strengths. (After Brange et al. 1982)

Table 19. Influence of zinc content in Actrapid (USP-formulation) on the relative physical stability. (Brange et al. 1986)

Zinc/hexamer	U 40	U 100	U 500
0	1	1.1	3.2
2	2.5	3	15
3		5	35
4	75	100	500

The marked fibrillation-inhibitory effect of increasing the zinc ion concentration from 2 Zn/hexamer to 4 Zn/hexamer (Brange and Havelund 1983c, Brange et al. 1986) is probably also due to a stabilizing effect on the hexamer (Table 19).

The more precise requirements to physical and chemical stability of insulins for use in pumps can only be defined when experience has been gained with the implantable devices presently under development.

XII. Insulin Derivatives

Numerous attempts have been made to modify the primary structure of insulin in an endeavour to: 1. gain more detailed knowledge of the spatial organization of the molecule and the role of the functional groups in stabilizing the secondary, tertiary and quaternary structure; 2. localize the biologically active part of the molecule in order to understand the molecular mechanisms of binding and action; 3. obtain analogues with a prolonged timing of action; 4. reduce the antigenicity and/or immunogenicity in therapeutic use. The first two aspects have been reviewed by Blundell et al. (1972) and Pullen et al. (1976) and will not be dealt with here.

An insulin analogue possessing a protracted effect was prepared for the first time by Hallas-Møller (1945), who coupled insulin with phenylisocyanate and found that the resulting phenylcarbamoyl insulin (Iso-insulin), although soluble at physiological pH, showed a slow onset and prolongation of effect. Iso-insulin and a mixture of Iso-insulin and regular insulin (Di-insulin) were in therapeutic use for many years, but have been withdrawn. Later Bradbury et al. (1973) prepared a series of reversible derivatives of insulin in an attempt to obtain a retarded action by changing the isoelectric point and lowering the solubility at tissue pH, but sufficiently long duration of action was not obtained.

Various modified insulins have been tried for the treatment of the rare cases of immunological insulin resistance, the objective being to reduce the affinity to insulin antibodies in the patient's serum. The successful use of des-alanine(B-30) porcine insulin was reported by Boshell et al. (1964), Kumar and Miller (1970), and Burman et al. (1973). The immunological significance of the B-chain carboxy-terminal amino acid (Ala B-30) was reviewed by Kumar (1979), who found that two thirds of diabetics resistant to insulin had antibodies differentiating between porcine and desalanine porcine insulin, with a lower affinity for the latter. The immunological properties of insulin analogues substituted at position B-30 by different amino acid residues have been investigated by Neubauer et al. (1984), who found that the individual analogues stimulated antibody development (immunogenicity) to the same extent as did the parent insulin, whereas the binding capacity to pre-formed antibodies (antigenicity) was reduced to 80–90% of that of the parent insulin.

However, desalanine (B-30) porcine insulin appears less efficacious when compared with sulphated insulin (Davidson and DeBra 1978). Sulphated insulin is a preparation containing porcine or bovine insulin treated with sulphuric acid (Moloney et al. 1964), resulting in a heterogenous mixture of at least nine different derivatives containing on average 4.5 sulphate ester groups per molecule.

The sulphation of beef insulin results in more than 50 percent loss of potency and 400 percent increase in cost (Little et al. 1977). Zeuzem et al. (1985) found that 22 times and 4 times the concentration of sulphated insulin was required to achieve equivalent biological effect in rat and human adipocytes, respectively. Pongor et al. (1983) using mild reaction conditions have prepared sulphated insulin with 2 sulphate groups per molecule and a bioactivity of about 80%. Successful treatment of insulin resistance has been reported by Maloney (1964), Menczel et al. (1966), and Little and Arnott (1966).

Des-phenylalanine insulin, which is an analogue obtained by removal of the N-terminal amino acid of the B-chain (Brandenburg 1969, Kerp et al. 1974) has been introduced in a variety of different formulations (Sachse et al. 1982). The immunogenicity of this derivative has been found to be comparable with native insulin of the same species, whereas the binding capacity to pre-existing antibodies seemed to be less than that of unmodified insulin (Santeusanio et al. 1981). Thus, Valdenaire and Klein (1979) treated 11 patients with insulin resistance and achieved a considerable decrease of insulin requirement in more than half of the patients. A clinical long-term trial (Hirn et al. 1982) and a comparative study with conventional preparations (Sachse and Federlin 1981), have not revealed significant clinical advantages of Des-Phe-preparations with respect to metabolic control.

Recently, the physiologic effects of human proinsulin, the biosynthetic precursor of human insulin (Steiner and Oyer 1967) and now available through recombinant DNA technology (cf. D.I), have been studied in normals and diabetic patients (Revers et al. 1984, Bergenstal et al. 1984, Glauber et al. 1986).

XIII. Alternative Administration of Insulin

The chemical character of insulin was not known during the first years after the discovery of the hormone and it was natural to try different ways of administration; therefore a number of parenteral as well as several non-parenteral routes, including cutaneous, nasal, lingual, tracheal, oral, intestinal, rectal and vaginal, were tested.

It soon became clear that insulin was administered most effectively by parenteral injection, but due to the discomfort and inconvenience of injection therapy a great many efforts were made to improve the non-parenteral administration forms by protecting the insulin molecule from enzymatic degradation and facilitating the absorption by addition of various substances. At least 60 reports were published during the first 15 years of insulin therapy (Jensen 1938), but all these attempts were without or with limited or varying success.

In recent years new formulation techniques have been used in attempt to develop dosage forms of insulin applicable for absorption by oral, nasal, rectal or other mucosal routes. Recent results are reviewed in the following.

Nasal absorption of insulin has been demonstrated in animals and humans. Hirai et al. found that the absorption through the nasal mucosa in dogs (1978) or in rats (1981) was promoted when a surfactant was present and showed that addition of 1% polyoxyethylene-9-lauryl ether or bile salts to the insulin solution resulted in a bioavailability of about 30% compared with intravenous administration. Using one of the same bile salts (sodium glycocholate) Pontiroli et al. (1982) found only about 10% bioavailability when insulin was given intranasally to normal subjects and diabetic patients and Hirata et. al. (1983) observed damage to the microvilli of the nasal mucous membrane upon repeated administration of sodium glycocholate. Compared with subcutaneous administration a more rapid increase in serum insulin concentration resulting in a prompt reduction of blood glucose concentration was seen with bile salt promoted nasal absorption in normal and diabetic subjects (Moses et al. 1983), but large differences in absorption were observed correlating positively with increasing hydrophobicity of the steroid nucleus of the bile salts (Gordon et al. 1985). Salzman et al. (1985) assessed the efficacy of 1% polyoxyethylene-9-lauryl ether in long-term studies in diabetics and found that the absorption profile more closely simulated that of endogenously secreted insulin in response to a meal than that of subcutaneously injected insulin, but less than 10% bioavailability was obtained compared with intravenous administration.

Absorption across *respiratory mucosae* on delivery of regular insulin by aerosol inhalation was reported in humans by Wigley et al. (1971), but only low and variable efficiency was obtained. Administered as powdered aerosol and delivered directly into the trachea of rabbits the bioavailability has been shown to be approx. 40% (Yoshida et al. 1979). Ishida et al. (1981) investigated the absorption through *oral mucosa* (buccal cavity) of dogs and found that the percentage of insulin absorbed from a new dosage form was about 0.5% compared with intramuscular injection of insulin.

A variety of different new formulations have been tested in order to increase the effectiveness of *oral* administration of insulin by use of surfactants, insulin derivatives, adsorption of insulin to small particles or entrapment of insulin in organic vehicles. These attempts include administration of insulin: 1. together with polyethylene-20-oleyl ether (Brij 98) to normals and diabetic patients (Galloway and Root 1972); 2. adsorbed physically on β-naphthyl-azo-polystyrene particles (Shichiri et al. 1971) or cross-linked with glutaraldehyde (Oppenheim et al. 1982) to rabbits and mice or rats, respectively; 3. entrapped in phosphatidyl choline liposomes (Dapergolas and Gregoriadis 1976, Tragl et al. 1979, and Arrieta-Molero et al. 1982) or in water-in-oil-in-water emulsions (Shichiri et al. 1976) to rats or rabbits. Only low and inconsistent efficiency ($\leq 1\%$ bioavailability) has been reported in these articles, and no dose response relationship was demonstrated.

Furthermore, the stability and effectiveness of liposome-entrapped insulin was unpredictable (Arrieta-Molero et al. 1982, Shenfield and Hill 1982).Using coating of insulin with polymers cross-linked with an azoaromatic group, Saffran et al. (1986) observed a certain blood sugar lowering effect in normal rats after oral administration, but the maximal responses occurred at variable times, from 1 to 9 hours after administration of the protected insulin.

Direct *intestinal* administration of insulin has been tried in a number of cases. Crane et al. (1968) showed that injected into the upper jejunum of a pancreatec- tomized man, the fraction of insulin absorbed did not exceed about 0.5% of the dose given in spite of the total absence of pancreatic proteolytic enzymes. Given together with absorption-promoting substances to diabetic rats the efficiency of intestinal absorption was 3–10% compared with parenteral administration (Shi- chiri et al. 1975, Touitou et al. 1980).

Rectal absorption of insulin formulated as suppositories prepared by mixing insulin with surfactants has been described by a number of groups. Shichiri et al. (1978) found the absorption in depancreatized dogs more rapid than after intra- muscular injection, but the comparative efficiency was only about 10%. Ichikawa et al. (1980) tested the absorption promoting effect in rabbits of a variety of non- ionic, anionic, cationic and amphoteric surfactants including bile acids and found an optimal effect of suppositories with 1% polyoxyethylene-9-lauryl ether. How- ever, the dose of rectally administered insulin needed to produce hypoglycaemia of similar magnitude was about two or three times the intravenous dose.

Using the same optimal surfactant, Yamasaki et al. investigated rectal appli- cation of insulin suppositories in diabetic dogs (1981 a) and in normal and dia- betic human subjects (1981 b). They found evidence that 30% of the insulin ab- sorbed from the rectum was distributed to the portal vein, but the total bioavail- ability was not more than about 10%. By rectal administration of microenema containing 5-methoxysalicylate Nishihata et al. (1983) found maximum plasma insulin levels in dogs after 45 minutes and a bioavailability of approximately 25% compared with i.m. administration. An increase of bioavailability from 19 to 38% compared with intramuscular administration was observed when the suppository with insulin plus adjuvant was followed by another suppository with adjuvant only (Nishihata et al. 1985). Using sodium salicylate as primary adjuvant Liversidge et al. (1985), after rectal administration in dogs, observed a greater decrease of blood glucose levels with increasing content of acetic acid in the suppository. Hildebrandt et al. (1984) found in diabetic patients approximately 5% uptake of insulin from suppositories containing Brij 58 compared with sub- cutaneous injection. Rectal administration of insulin has been reviewed by Ritschel and Ritschel (1984) who also discussed the pharmacological aspects of rectal insulin absorption.

Thus, even by use of modern application forms the nonparenteral routes of administration of insulin have not so far resulted in reliable alternatives to the parenteral routes.

In recent years new approaches have been suggested for parenteral insulin de- livery. These include subcutaneous implantation in rats of small vinyl-ethylene copolymer pellets (Creque et al. 1980, Brown et al. 1986) or biodegradable insulin-albumin microbeads (Goosen et al. 1983), which can release insulin at constant rate for several weeks, and intravenous injection of maltose-insulin derivatives bound to lectin in complexes which allow displacement of varying amounts of hormone when exposed to glucose solutions of different concentrations (Brownlee and Cerami 1979, 1983, Sato et al. 1984). The clinical usefulness of these approaches remains, however, to be seen.

D. Human Insulin

I. Manufacture

1. Sources

Human insulin has been prepared from four sources:

a) From human pancreas. The amount of human insulin that can be prepared from cadaveric pancreas glands is totally inadequate for therapy.

b) From amino acids by peptide synthesis (Sieber et al. 1974, 1977). The 200 reaction steps of a total synthesis make the product extremely costly.

c) From porcine insulin by a semisynthetic conversion into human insulin. Porcine insulin can be made in sufficient quantities to meet the demands for the next decades and a quantitative conversion process for large-scale production has been developed (cf. D.I.2).

d) From fermentation of E. coli bacteria or Saccharomyces cerevisiae yeast, suitably encoded by DNA recombinant methods. This source is, in theory, unlimited (cf. D.I.3).

The methods relevant for the manufacture of human insulin are c) developed by NOVO and d) developed by E. Lilly (E. coli) and later by NOVO (Saccharomyces cerevisiae). Sources and characteristics of human insulins of different origin have been reviewed by Ege (1985).

2. Conversion of Porcine Insulin

Porcine insulin is converted to an ester of human insulin in a transpeptidation reaction, in which the alanine residue No. 30 of the B-chain is replaced by a threonine ester. The reaction is catalysed by porcine trypsin and takes place in a mixture of water and organic solvents in the presence of a large excess of the threonine ester (Markussen 1980, Markussen 1982, Markussen and Schaumburg 1983). The reaction mechanism is depicted in Fig. 32. First, porcine insulin and trypsin associate under formation of the Michaelis complex. Then the alanine residue (Ala^{B30}) is split off under formation of des(Ala^{B30})-insulinyl-trypsin ester, (DAI – trypsin), the ester being formed from the carboxyl group of lysine (Lys^{B29}) and the hydroxyl group of serine (Ser^{183}) in the active site of trypsin.

Hydrolysis of this intermediate is suppressed in the reaction medium, and instead the threonine ester brings about an aminolysis rendering the human insulin ester, first as the Michaelis complex which eventually dissociates. The yield of hu-

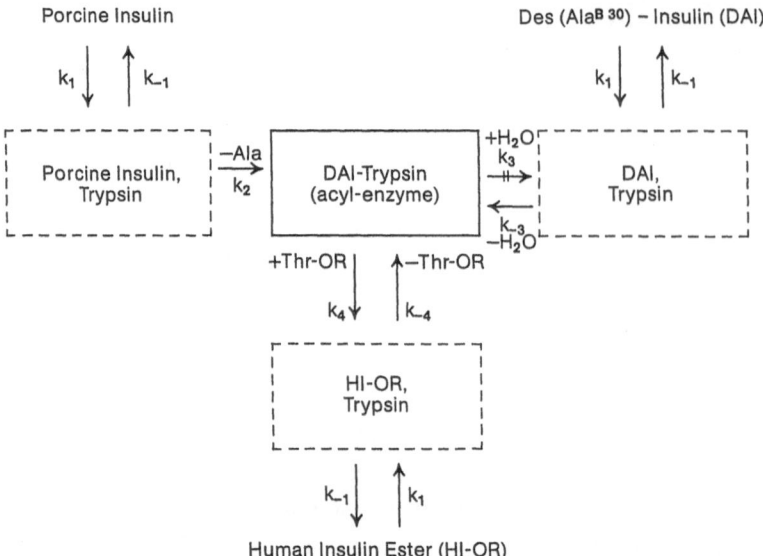

Fig. 32. Reaction mechanism of the trypsin catalyzed transpeptidation of porcine insulin into human insulin ester. Michaelis complexes are in *boxes with broken lines*. The uptake of water (k_3) under formation of desalanine insulin (*DAI*) is suppressed in the reaction medium. (Markussen et al. 1982)

man insulin ester in the transpeptidation reaction is about 97%. Proinsulin and related compounds present in crude insulin are likewise transpeptidized to human insulin ester, thus making a contribution to the yield of about 3%.

The further processing to human monocomponent insulin is shown in Fig. 33 (Markussen 1982, Markussen et al. 1982). Trypsin is removed by column chromatography at a low pH where it is inactive. Residual amounts of unconverted porcine insulin are removed by anion exchange chromatography. As porcine insulin contains an additional negative charge relative to the human insulin ester, the product is the first to emerge from the column. The ester group is cleaved rendering human insulin. A final ion exchange chromatography removes any residual human insulin ester and ensures that the final product fulfills the specifications for the monocomponent insulins. The data and purity tests of relevance to human insulin originating from porcine insulin are compiled in the second column of Table 20.

3. Biosynthesis in E. coli

The strategy developed for biosynthesis of human insulin is depicted in Fig. 34 (Goeddel et al. 1979, Chance et al. 1981 a–c). DNA sequences encoding for the A and B chains of insulin were synthesized chemically. A codon for methionine was introduced at the N-terminals of the A and B chain genes. The tryptophan synthetase operon, trp E, was placed in front of the methionine codon, and the two constructed genes were inserted into plasmids and cloned separately in E. coli. Fermentations of the bacteria containing the plasmids result in the pro-

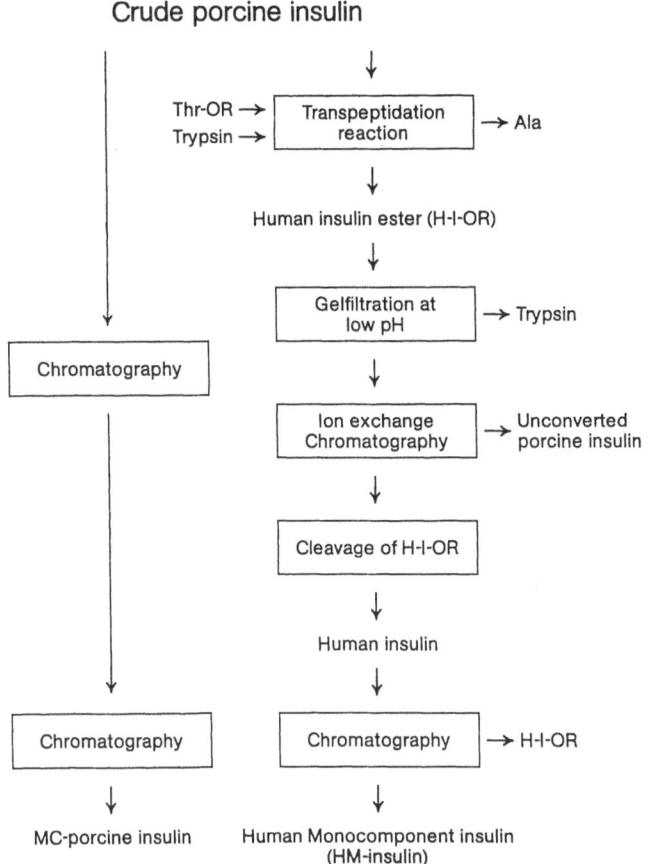

Fig. 33. Flow sheet of the production of Human Monocomponent insulin from crude porcine insulin. (After Markussen et al. 1982)

duction of chimeric proteins consisting of a tryptophan synthetase fragment followed by methionine and either the A or the B chain. The large chimeric proteins precipitate in the cytoplasm of E. coli, the precipitation thus preventing proteolysis of the insulin chains by the proteases of the cytoplasm. The chimeric protein amounts to 20% of the total protein in the cells and a yield of 10^5 molecules per cell can be achieved (Goeddel et al. 1979).

After the fermentations the cells are harvested and the chimeric proteins are isolated from the cells. The insulin chains are released from the chimeric partner by treatment with cyanogen bromide, which specifically cleaves at methionine residues, Fig. 34. This cleavage is possible since human insulin has no methionine residues. The methionine residues are converted into homoserine residues still attached to the tryptophan synthetase fragment.

The insulin chains are then converted to the S-sulphonates, which are easy to handle and purify in aqueous solution. The next step is the critical chain combi-

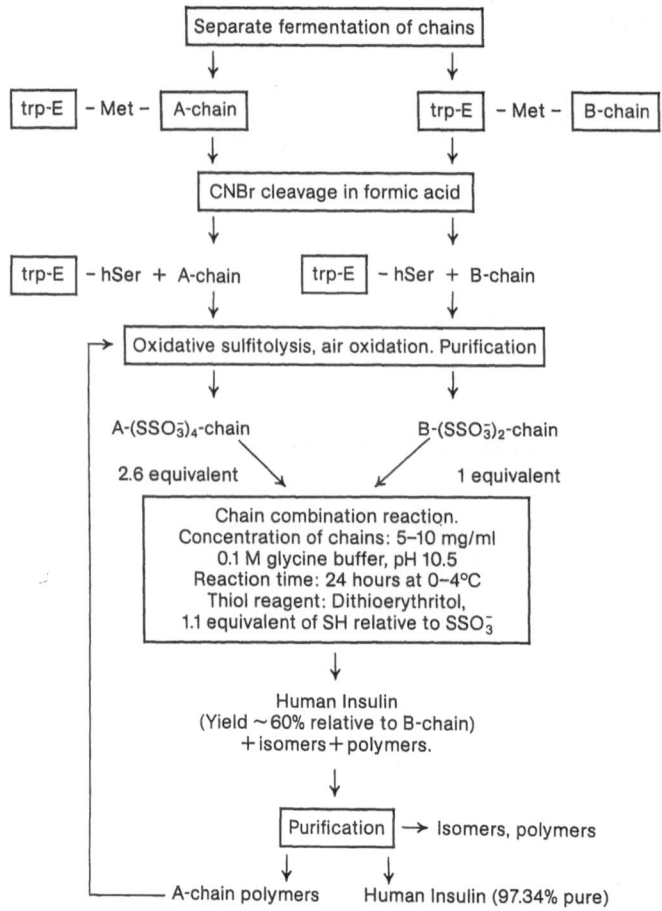

Fig. 34. Flow sheet of the production of human insulin from the fermentations of the insulin chains in separate clones of E. coli. Purity according to Chance et al. (1981 b). *Met* methionine; *h-Ser* homoserine; *CNBr* cyanogen bromide; *trp E* tryptophansynthetase E

nation reaction. From one A-chain and one B-chain it is, in theory, possible to form 12 isomeric compounds, only one of which is insulin.

By applying an exchange reaction between S-sulphonates and thiols (Chance et al. 1981 c) conditions were found that yielded satisfactory yields of insulin, cf. Fig. 34.

The reactions are formally:

$$A-SSO_3^- + R(SH)_2 \rightarrow A-SH + R\overset{SH}{\underset{SSO_3^-}{\diagdown}} \rightarrow R\overset{S}{\underset{S}{\diagup}} + HSO_3^-$$

$$A-SH + B-SSO_3^- \rightarrow A-S-S-B + HSO_3^-$$

$$HSO_3^- + OH^- \rightarrow H_2O + SO_3^-.$$

Table 20. Data and purity tests of the two human insulins, originating from porcine pancreatic glands and fermentation of E. coli bacteria, respectively

Origin	Porcine insulin	E. coli bacteria
Manufacturer	Novo	E. Lilly
Potency of dry substance	28.5 ± 0.8 IU/mg	27.5 ± 1.7 IU/mg
Method of bioassay	Mouse convulsion	Rabbit hypoglycemia
Purity by HPLC[a]	>99%	>97%
Porcine insulin	n.d., d.l. <0.1%	–
Porcine PLI[b]	<1 ppm	–
Porcine trypsin	$<1:10^{22}$ (w/w)	–
"E. coli proteins", RIA[c]	–	<4 ppm[e]
Endotoxin, LAL[d] test	–	<0.6 ppm

[a] High pressure liquid chromatography
[b] Proinsulin like immunoreactivity
[c] Radio immunoassay
[d] Limulus amebocyte lysate
[e] Quantitation of a heterogeneous contamination dependent upon antiserum and standard.
Abbreviations: n.d. non-detectable; d.l. detection limit

After purification, i.e. removal of isomers and polymers, human insulin with a purity of about 97% is obtained (Chance et al. 1981 b). Data and purity tests indicative for human insulin produced in E. coli are compiled in the third column of Table 20. The E. coli protein contaminants have been estimated by a RIA and four batches contained less than 1 ppm, while detectable amounts (3.3 ppm) were found in one batch (Baker et al. 1981). It must, however, be realized that attempting to quantify the heterogenous mixtures of E. coli contaminants as a single value by RIA poses certain problems, as the results may vary dependent on the antisera, tracer and standard used, as well as on the composition of the sample.

More recently a process using DNA sequences encoding for human proinsulin has been described for production of human insulin in E. coli (Frank et al. 1981). The fermentation steps in this method are in principle similar to the steps described for the A- and B-chain biosynthesis, but the post-fermentation chemistry is simpler as the chain combination process now is directed by the proinsulin C-peptide.

4. Biosynthesis in Saccharomyces cerevisiae

An alternative method of manufacture of human insulin by biosynthesis in yeast has recently been described (Markussen et al. 1986a, b, Thim et al. 1986).

Recombinant plasmids coding for single-chain insulin precursors with only a few amino acid residues linking the A- and B-chain are inserted into a S. cerevisiae strain, which is grown in continuous fermentation. During fermentation the single-chain insulin precursor is exported to the broth with free B-chain N-terminal and with the correct disulfide bridges formed. After removal of yeast cells, it is isolated from the broth by adsorption on an ion exchange column. The precursor is converted by tryptic transpeptidation to a double-chain human insulin ester, followed by hydrolysis of the ester, a process similar to the conversion of porcine to human insulin (cf. D.I.2). Purification including 2 crystallizations, gel filtration, 2 anion chromatographies and a final purification by HPLC resulted in a purity of 99.5–99.9% as assessed by analytical HPLC. Yeast protein contaminants were detected to be less than 1 ppm (detection limit 1 ppm) by an ELISA method (Markussen et al. 1986a, b).

II. Preparations

The availability of human insulin in large quantities has resulted in the introduction of several different pharmaceutical preparations covering the need for short-, intermediate- and long-acting types. In principle the formulations of these human insulin preparations with respect to content of auxilliary substances (cf. C.V) and mechanisms of prolongation (cf. C.II.6, C.IV) are the same as those of their porcine or bovine counterparts.

It has been observed that the regular human insulins are absorbed somewhat quicker than porcine insulin, irrespective of the source and brand of the human insulin (Federlin et al. 1981, Cüppers et al. 1982, Owens 1986). This quicker absorption might be due to the fact that human insulin is more hydrophilic than porcine insulin, but a tendency to less association of human insulin into hexamers than that of porcine insulin, as revealed in a gel filtration experiment (Brange, unpublished), can also be a possible explanation.

The same tendency of a quicker initial effect of human intermediate- and long-acting preparations has also been observed when compared with the corresponding porcine or bovine formulations. Thus, a quicker initial effect and shorter duration of action of NPH made from biosynthetic human insulin than porcine NPH have been reported (Enzmann at al. 1982, Clark et al. 1982, Owens et al. 1984). In contrast to these results, Hildebrandt et al. (1984) found no difference between absorption rate of NPH insulins from different species when given in equal doses but observed a relatively lower absorption rate for a large than for a small dose. Monotard HM was not different from the porcine Monotard MC in a short-term, double-blind, cross-over study (Sestoft et al. 1982) nor in longer, open switch-over studies (Egstrup and Olsen 1982, Vestermark 1982). In a fifteen-month double-blind crossover study Home et al. (1984) found a small, but clinically significant, pharmacokinetic difference between human and porcine insulin in patients treated with Actrapid and Monotard.

Human Ultralente (Ultratard HM) was studied in a double blind crossover study in 18 diabetics and found as effective as bovine Ultralente in controlling basal plasma glucose concentrations (Holman et al. 1984). Hildebrandt et al. (1985) reported a substantially faster absorption of human than bovine Ultralente, but concluded that human Ultralente is suitable as the basal insulin preparation for multiple insulin injection regimens. The faster absorption of the human relative to bovine Ultralente was confirmed by Owens et al. (1986). Clinical and pharmacological studies of human insulin have recently been reviewed by Owens (1986).

Immungenicity studies (cf. B.III) have shown that human MC insulin induced significantly less insulin antibodies than porcine MC insulin (Fankhauser et al.

1982, Schernthaner et al. 1983, Heding et al. 1984, Luyckx et al. 1986) and this may have clinical implications, as even small amounts of antibodies are associated with a reduced C-peptide secretion and a higher insulin requirement after about one year of insulin treatment of insulin-dependent diabetic children (Ludvigsson 1984, Schernthaner et al. 1984).

Introducing pure human insulin for the treatment of diabetes has finally made it possible to substitute diabetics' lack of endogenous insulin with an identical molecule.

References

Aaby P (1979) Concentration of porcine proinsulin-like material in plasma of insulin-treated diabetics in relation to purity of insulin preparations. Horm Metab Res 11:455–457

Abel JJ (1926) Crystalline insulin. Proc Natl Acad Sci (Wash) 12:132–136

Adams MJ, Blundell TL, Dodson EJ, Dodson GG, Vijayan M, Baker EN, Harding MM, Hodgkin DC, Rimmer B, Sheat S (1969) Structure of rhombohedral 2 zinc insulin crystals. Nature 224:491–495

Alameda GK, Evelhoch JL, Sudmeier JL, Birge RR (1985) Characterization of the internal calcium(II) binding sites in dissolved insulin hexamer using europium(III) fluorescence. Biochemistry 24:1757–1762

Albisser AM, Leibel BS, Ewart TG, Davidovac Z, Botz CK, Zingg W (1974) An artificial endocrine pancreas. Diabetes 23:389–396

Albisser AM, Lougheed W, Perlman K, Bahoric A (1980) Nonaggregating insulin solutions for long-term glucose control in experimental and human diabetes. Diabetes 29:241–243

Albisser AM, Lougheed WD, Chow JC, Tung AK (1982) A modified insulin for pumps. Diabetes 31 (Suppl. 2, part 2):67A (abstract)

Allwood MC (1978) Antimicrobial agents in single- and multi-dose injections. J Appl Bacteriol 44:Svii–Sxviii

Allwood MC (1982) The effectiveness of preservatives in insulin injections. Pharm J 229:340

Amaya FJ, Lee T-C, Chichester CO (1976) Biological inactivation of proteins by the Maillard reaction. Effect of mild heat on the tertiary structure of insulin. J Agric Food Chem 24:465–467

American Diabetes Association (1985) Policy statement, continuous subcutaneous insulin infusion. Diabetes 34:946–947

Andersen OO (1973) Insulin antibody formation. II The influence of species difference and method of administration. Acta Endocrinol 72:33–45

Ando T, Watanabe S (1969) A new method for fractionation of protamines and the amino acid sequences of salmine and three components of iridine. Int J Protein Res 1:221–224

Arnott RD, Cameron MA, Stepanas TV, Cohen M (1982) Insulin syringes. Dangers of dead space. Med J Aust 2:39–40

Arrieta-Molero JF, Aleck K, Sinha MK, Brownscheidle CM, Shapiro LJ, Sperling MA (1982) Orally administered liposome-entrapped insulin in diabetic animals. A critical assessment. Horm Res 16:249–256

Ashford WR, Campbell J, Davidson JK, Fisher AM, Haist RE, Lacey AH, Lin B, Martin JM, Morley NH, Rastogi KS, Storvick WO (1969) A consideration of methods of insulin assay. Diabetes 18:828–833

Baker RS, Schmidtke JR, Ross JW, Smith WC (1981) Preliminary studies on the immunogenicity and amounts of Escherichia coli polypeptides in biosynthetic human insulin produced by recombinant DNA technology. Lancet 2:1139–1142

Bang HO (1946) Some investigations on the absorption mechanism of protamine insulin. Acta Pharmacol Toxicol (Copenh) 2:79–88

Bangham DR, Mussett MV (1959) The fourth international standard for insulin. Bull WHO 20:1209–1220

Bangham DR, Jonge H de, Noordwijk J van (1978) The collaborative assay of the European pharmacopoeia biological reference preparation for insulin. J Biol Stand 6:301–314

Banting FG, Best CH (1922) Pancreatic extracts. J Lab Clin Med 7:464–472

Bentley G, Dodson E, Dodson G, Hodgkin D, Mercola D (1976) Structure of insulin in 4-zinc insulin. Nature 261:166–168

Bentley G, Dodson G, Lewitova A (1978) Rhombohedral insulin crystal transformation. J Mol Biol 126:871–875

Bergenstal RM, Cohen RM, Lever E, Polonsky K, Jaspan J, Blix PM, Revers R, Olefsky JM, Kolterman O, Steiner K, Cherrington A, Frank B, Galloway J, Rubenstein AH (1984) The metabolic effects of biosynthetic human proinsulin in individuals with type I diabetes. J Clin Endocrinol Metab 58:973–979

Berger M, Cüppers HJ, Hegner H, Jörgens V, Berchtold P (1982) Absorption kinetics and biologic effects of subcutaneously injected insulin preparations. Diabetes Care 5:77–91

Berger W, Keller U, Vorster D (1981) Verlauf und Therapie des Coma diabeticum. Internist (Berlin) 22:219–228

Bergman N, Vella ID (1982) Potential life-threatening variations of drug concentrations in intravenous infusion systems. Potassium chloride, insulin, and heparin. Med J Aust 2:270–272

Berson SA, Yalow RS (1959) Quantitative aspects of the reaction between insulin and insulin-binding antibody. J Clin Invest 38:1996–2016

Berson SA, Yalow RS (1960) Insulin inhibitors and insulin resistance. NY State J Med 60:3658–3665

Berson SA, Yalow RS (1964) The present status of insulin antagonists in plasma. Diabetes 13:247–259

Berson SA, Yalow RS, Bauman A, Rothschild MA, Newerly K (1956) Insulin-I^{131} metabolism in human subjects: Demonstration of insulin binding globulin in the circulation of insulin treated subjects. J Clin Invest 35:170–190

Bi RC, Dauter Z, Dodson E, Dodson G, Giordano F, Reynolds C (1984) Insulin's structure as a modified and monomeric molecule. Biopolymers 23:391–395

Biemond MEF, Sipman WA, Olivié J (1979) Quantitative determination of polypeptides by gradient elution high pressure liquid chromatography. J Liq Chromatogr 2:1407–1435

Binder C (1969) Absorption of injected insulin. Acta Pharmacol Toxicol (Copenh) (Suppl. 2) 27:1–87

Binder C, Nielsen AA, Jørgensen K (1967) The absorption of an acid and a neutral insulin solution after subcutaneous injection into different regions in diabetic patients. Scand J Clin Lab Invest 19:156–163

Birdi KS (1973) The binding of cationic detergent to insulin, zinc-insulin and Iso-insulin. Biochem J 135:253–255

Blackshear PJ, Rohde TD, Palmer JL, Wigness BD, Rupp WM, Buchwald H (1983) Glycerol prevents insulin precipitation and interruption of flow in an implantable insulin infusion pump. Diabetes Care 6:387–392

Blaug SM, Grant DE (1974) Kinetics of degradation of the parabens. J Soc Cosmet Chem 25:495–506

Bloom SR (1979) Vasoactive intestinal peptide. In: Jaffe BM, Behrman HR (eds) Methods of hormone radioimmunoassay. Academic Press, New York, pp 553–565

Bloom SR, West AM, Polak JM, Barnes AJ, Adrian TE (1978) Hormonal contaminants of insulin. In: Bloom SR (ed) Gut hormones. Churchill Livingstone, Edinburgh London New York, pp 318–322

Bloom SR, Barnes AJ, Adrian TE, Polak JM (1979) Autoimmunity in diabetics induced by hormonal contaminants of insulin. Lancet I:14–17

Blundell TL, Cutfield JF, Cutfield SM, Dodson EJ, Dodson GG, Hodgkin DC, Mercola DA, Vijayan M (1971) Atomic positions in rhombohedral 2-zinc insulin crystals. Nature 231:506–511

Blundell T, Dodson G, Hodgkin D, Mercola D (1972) Insulin: The structure in the crystal and its reflection in chemistry and biology. Adv Protein Chem 26:279–402

Boshell BR, Barrett JC, Wilensky AS, Patton TB (1964) Insulin resistance. Response to insulin from various animal sources, including human. Diabetes 13:144–152

Bottermann P, Hügler P, Schweigart U, Zilker T, Giebeler K, Enzmann F (1980) Ermittlung von Insulin-Wirkprofilen mit Hilfe des „Glukose-kontrollierten Insulin-Infusions-Systems" (Biostator®). Akt Endokrin 1:337–345

Bradbury AF, Ko ASC, Massey DE, Salokangas A, Smyth DG, Sabey GA, Webb FW, Stewart GA (1973) The quest for a latent action insulin. Postgrad Med J 49 (Suppl):945–948

Bradbury JH, Ramesh V, Dodson G (1981) ^{1}H nuclear magnetic resonance study of the histidine residues of insulin. J Mol Biol 150:609–613

Brandenburg D (1969) Des-Phe^{B1}-insulin, ein kristallines Analogon des Rinderinsulins. Hoppe-Seyler's Z Physiol Chem 350:741–750

Brange J, Havelund S (1983a) Properties of insulin in solution. In: Brunetti P, Alberti KGMM, Albisser AM, Hepp KD, Benedetti MM (eds) Artificial systems for insulin delivery. Raven Press, New York, pp 83–88

Brange J, Havelund S (1983b) Insulin pumps and insulin quality: Requirements and problems. Acta Med Scand (Suppl) 671:135–138

Brange J, Havelund S (1983c) Stabilized insulin preparations. US Patent 4476118

Brange J, Havelund S, Hansen P, Langkjær L, Sørensen E, Hildebrandt P (1982) Formulation of physically stable neutral insulin solution for continuous infusion by delivery systems. In: Gueriguian JL, Bransome ED, Outschoorn AS (eds) Hormone Drugs. United States Pharmacopeial Convention, Rockville, Maryland, pp 96–105

Brange J, Langkjær L, Havelund S, Sørensen E (1983) Chemical stability of insulin: Neutral insulin solutions. Diabetologia 25:193 (abstract)

Brange J, Langkjær L, Havelund S, Sørensen E (1984) Chemical stability of insulin: formation of covalent insulin dimers and other higher molecular weight transformation products in intermediate- and long-acting insulin preparations. Diabetologia 27:259A–260A (abstract)

Brange J, Langkjær L, Havelund S, Sørensen E (1985) Chemical stability of insulin: formation of desamido insulins and other hydrolytic products in intermediate and long acting insulin preparations. Diabetes Res Clin Pract (Suppl 1) p 67 (abstract)

Brange J, Havelund S, Hommel E, Sørensen E, Kühl C (1986) Neutral insulin solutions physically stabilized by addition of Zn^{2+}. Diabetic Medicine 3:532–536

Brange J, Hansen JF, Havelund S, Melberg SG (1987) Studies of the insulin fibrillation process. In: Brunetti P, Waldhäusl W (eds) Advanced models for the therapy of insulin-dependent diabetes. Raven Press, New York, pp 85–90

Brill AS, Venable JH (1968) The binding of transition metal ions in insulin crystals. J Mol Biol 36:343–353

Bringer J, Heldt A, Grodsky GM (1981) Prevention of insulin aggregation by dicarboxylic amino acids during prolonged infusion. Diabetes 30:83–85

British Pharmacopoeia (1980) vol I+II. Her Majesty's Stationery Office, London

Brown L, Munoz C, Siemer L, Edelman E, Langer R (1986) Controlled release of insulin from polymer matrices. Control of diabetes in rats. Diabetes 35:692–697

Browne M, Cecil R, Miller JC (1973) Some reactions of insulin at non-polar surfaces. Eur J Biochem 33:233–240

Brownlee M, Cerami A (1979) A glucose-controlled insulin-delivery system: Semisynthetic insulin bound to lectin. Science 206:1190–1191

Brownlee M, Cerami A (1983) Glycosylated insulin complexed to concanavalin A. Biochemical basis for a closed-loop insulin delivery system. Diabetes 32:499–504

Brunfeldt K, Poulsen JE (1953) Protamine-splitting enzyme from serum and subcutaneous tissue. Rep Steno Mem Hosp Nord Insulinlab 5:51–61

Buchwald H, Rohde TD, Dorman FD, Skakoon JG, Wigness BD, Prosl FR, Tucker EM, Rublein TG, Blackshear PJ, Varco RL (1980) A totally implantable drug infusion device: Laboratory and clinical experience using a model with single flow rate and new design for modulated insulin infusion. Diabetes Care 3:351–358

Buchwald H, Varco RL, Rupp WM, Goldenberg FJ, Barbosa J, Rohde TD, Schwartz RA, Rublein TG, Blackshear PJ (1981) Treatment of a type II diabetic by a totally implantable insulin infusion device. Lancet I:1233–1235

Burgermeister W, Enzmann F, Schöne H-H (1975) The isolation of insulin from the pancreas. In: Hasselblatt A, Bruchhausen F von (eds) Insulin. Handbook of Experimental Pharmacology, vol XXXII/2. Springer, Berlin Heidelberg New York, pp 715–727

Burke MJ, Rougvie MA (1972) Cross-β protein structures. I. Insulin fibrils. Biochemistry 11:2435–2439

Burman KD, Cunningham EJ, Klachko DM, Burns TW (1973) Successful treatment of insulin resistance with dealaninated pork insulin (DPI). Mo Med 70:363–366

Caplan SN, Berkman EM (1976) Protamine sulfate and fish allergy. N Engl J Med 295:172

Carpenter FH (1958) Partition column chromatography of insulin in 2-butanol-aqueous acid systems. Arch Biochem Biophys 78:539–545

Carpenter FH (1966) Relationship of structure to biological activity of insulin as revealed by degradative studies. Am J Med 40:750–758

Cavallini D, Federici G, Barboni E, Marcucci M (1970) Formation of persulfide groups in alkaline treated insulin. FEBS Lett 10:125–128

Caygill CPJ, Ayling CM (1979) Effect of contaminating proteolytic activity upon insulin and insulin-protamine complex. J Pharm Pharmacol 31:849–852

Chan Y-K, Oda G, Kaplan H (1981) Chemical properties of the functional groups of insulin. Biochem J 193:419–425

Chance RE (1972) Amino acid sequences of proinsulins and intermediates. Diabetes 21 (Suppl 2):461–467

Chance RE, Ellis RM, Bromer WW (1968) Porcine proinsulin: Characterization and amino acid sequence. Science 161:165–167

Chance RE, Root MA, Galloway JA (1976) The immunogenicity of insulin preparations. Acta Endocrinol (Suppl 205) (Copenh) 83:185–196

Chance RE, Moon NE, Johnson MG (1979) Human pancreatic polypeptide (HPP) and bovine pancreatic polypeptide (BPP). In: Jaffe BM, Behrman HR (eds) Methods of hormone radioimmunoassay. Academic Press, New York, pp 657–672

Chance RE, Kroeff EP, Hoffmann JA (1981 a) Chemical, physical, and biological properties of recombinant human insulin. In: Gueriguian JL (ed) Insulins, growth hormone, and recombinant DNA technology. Raven Press, New York, pp 71–86

Chance RE, Kroeff EP, Hoffmann JA, Frank BH (1981 b) Chemical, physical and biological properties of biosynthetic human insulin. Diabetes Care 4:147–154

Chance RE, Hoffmann JA, Kroeff EP, Johnson MG, Schirmer EW, Bromer WW (1981 c) The production of human insulin using recombinant DNA technology and a new chain combination procedure. In: Rick DH, Gross E (eds) Peptides: Synthesis-Structure-Function. Proceedings of the seventh American peptide symposium. Pierce Chemical Company, Rockford, Illinois, pp 721–728

Chasteen ND, DeKoch RJ, Rogers BL, Hanna MW (1973) Use of vanadyl (IV) ion as a new spectroscopic probe of metal binding to proteins. Vanadyl insulin. J Am Chem Soc 95:1301–1309

Chawdhury SA, Dodson EJ, Dodson GG, Reynolds CD, Tolley SP, Blundell TL, Cleasby A, Pitts JE, Tickle IJ, Wood SP (1983) The crystal structures of three non-pancreatic human insulins. Diabetologia 25:460–464

Chothia C, Lesk AM, Dodson GG, Hodgkin DC (1983) Transmission of conformational change in insulin. Nature 302:500–505

Clark AJL, Knight G, Wiles PG, Keen H, Ward JD, Cauldwell JM, Adeniyi-Jones RO, Leiper JM, Jones RH, MacCuish AC, Watkins PJ, Glynne A, Scotton JB (1982) Biosynthetic human insulin in the treatment of diabetes. Lancet 2:354–357

Cogswell JJ, Simpson RM (1980) Introduction of U-100 insulin. Br Med J 280:566

Colagiuri S, Villalobos S (1986) Assessing effect of mixing insulins by glucose-clamp technique in subjects with diabetes mellitus. Diabetes Care 9:579–586

Cole RD (1960) The chromatography of insulin in urea-containing buffer. J Biol Chem 235:2294–2299

Colwell AR (1947) Protamine insulin mixtures in the treatment of diabetes mellitus. NY State J Med 47:1103–1110

Corran PH, Waley SG (1975) The reaction of penicillin with proteins. Biochem J 149:357–364

Crane CW, Path MC, Luntz GRWN (1986) Absorption of insulin from the human small intestine. Diabetes 17:625–627

Creque HM, Langer R, Folkman J (1980) One month of sustained release of insulin from a polymer implant. Diabetes 29:37–40

Cunningham LW, Fischer RL, Vestling CS (1955) A study of the binding of zinc and cobalt by insulin. J Am Chem Soc 77:5703–5707

Cüppers HJ, Franzke D, Esken P, Jörgens V, Berger M (1982) Pharmakokinetik und biologische Aktivität von semisynthetischen und biosynthetischen Humaninsulin-Präparaten. Aktuel Endokrinol Stoffwechsel 3:102

Damgaard U, Kruse V (1982) Inherent problems in radioimmunoassay exemplified by determination of proinsulin-like immunoreactivity in bovine insulin. In: Gueriguian JL, Bransome ED, Outschoorn AS (eds) Hormone Drugs. United States Pharmacopeial Convention, Rockville, Maryland, pp 187–191

Damgaard U, Markussen J (1979) Analysis of insulins and related compounds by HPLC. Horm Metab Res 11:580–581

Dapergolas G, Gregoriadis G (1976) Hypoglycaemic effect of liposome-entrapped insulin administered intragastrically into rats. Lancet II:824–827

Davidson JK, DeBra DW (1978) Immunologic insulin resistance. Diabetes 27:307–318

Davis BJ (1964) Disc electrophoresis – II. Ann NY Acad Sci 121:404–427

Diezel W, Kopperschläger G, Hofmann E (1972) An improved procedure for protein staining in polyacrylamide gels with a new type of Coomassie Brilliant Blue. Anal Biochem 48:617–620

Dinner A, Lorenz L (1979) High performance liquid chromatographic determination of bovine insulin. Anal Chem 51:1872–1873

Dodson E, Harding MM, Hodgkin DC, Rossmann MG (1966) The crystal structure of insulin. III. Evidence for a 2-fold axis in rhombohedral zinc insulin. J Mol Biol 16:227–241

Dodson EJ, Dodson GG, Lewitova A, Sabesan M (1978) Zinc-free cubic pig insulin: Crystallization and structure determination. J Mol Biol 125:387–396

Dodson EJ, Dodson GG, Hodgkin DC, Reynolds CD (1979) Structural relationships in the two-zinc insulin hexamer. Can J Biochem 57:469–479

Dörzbach E von, Müller R (1971) Die Insulintherapie: Die Insulinpräparate. In: Pfeiffer EF (Hrsg) Handbook of Diabetes Mellitus. Pathophysiology and clinical considerations. Vol. II. J. F. Lehmann's Verlag, München, pp 1087–1111

Dunn MF, Pattison SE, Storm MC, Quiel E (1980) Comparison of the zinc binding domains in the 7 S nerve growth factor and the zinc-insulin hexamer. Biochemistry 19:718–725

Easter BRD, Sutton DA, Drewes SE (1978) Crystalline (A21-desamido) bovine insulin. Hoppe-Seyler's Z Physiol Chem 359:1229–1236

Ege H (1985) Sources and characteristics of the human insulins. In: Breimer DD, Speiser P (eds) Topics in pharmaceutical sciences. Elsevier Science Publishers B.V., Amsterdam New York Oxford, pp 57–70

Ege H (1986) Semantics of insulin. Diabetic Medicine 3:212–215

Egstrup K , Olsen J (1982) Treatment with human insulin in outpatient diabetics. Lancet II:222–223

Ellenbogen E (1949) The determination of the physical-chemical properties of insulin and their application to the equilibrium between insulin of molecular weights 12,000 and 36,000. Dissertation, Harvard University

Emdin SO, Dodson GG, Cutfield JM, Cutfield SM (1980) Role of zinc in insulin biosynthesis. Some possible zinc-insulin interactions in the pancreatic B-cell. Diabetologia 19:174–182

Eneroth G, Aahlund K (1968) Biological assay of insulin by blood sugar determination in mice. Acta Pharm Suec 5:591–594

Eneroth G, Aahlund K (1970a) A twin cross-over method for bioassay of insulin using blood glucose levels in mice – a comparison with a rabbit method. Acta Pharm Suec 7:457–462

Eneroth G, Aahlund K (1970b) Exogenous insulin and blood glucose levels in mice. Acta Pharm Suec 7:491–500

Enzmann F, Balikcioglu S, Glynne A, Scotton J, Marsden J (1982) Zusammenfassende Betrachtung der klinischen Erprobung von Biosynthetischem Human-Insulin in Europa. In: Petersen KG, Schlüter KJ, Kerp L (Hrsg) Neue Insuline. Freiburger Graphische Betriebe, Freiburg, pp 181–186

European Pharmacopoeia (1975) III Council of Europe (European Treaty Series No. 50) Maisonneuve S.A., Sainte-Ruffine, p 78

Fahrenkrug J, Schaffalitzky de Muckadell OB (1977) Radioimmunoassay of vasoactive intestinal polypeptide (VIP) in plasma. J Lab Clin Med 89:1379–1388

Falholt K (1982) Determination of insulin specific IgE in serum of diabetic patients by solid-phase radioimmunoassay. Diabetologia 22:254–257

Falholt K, Hoskam JAM, Karamanos BG, Süsstrunk H, Viswanathan M, Heding LG (1983) Insulin-specific IgE in serum of 67 diabetic patients against human insulin (Novo), porcine insulin, and bovine insulin. Four case reports. Diabetes Care 6:61–65

Fankhauser S, Herz G, Zuppinger K (1982) Expérience avec l'insuline humaine chez des enfants diabétiques. Med Hyg 40:1378–1384

Federlin K, Laube H, Velcovsky HG (1981) Biologic and immunologic in vivo and in vitro studies with biosynthetic human insulin. Diabetes Care 4:170–174

Feingold V, Jenkins AB, Kraegen EW (1984) Effect of contact material on vibration-induced insulin aggregation. Diabetologia 27:373–378

Finger H, Schaeg W, Niemann H (1967) Untersuchungen über den Einfluß von überschüssigem Zink auf die Aggregation von nativem und photooxidiertem Insulin. Experientia 23:435

Fisher BV, Porter PB (1981) Stability of bovine insulin. J Pharm Pharmacol 33:203–206

Fisher BV, Smith D (1986) HPLC as a replacement for the animal response assays for insulin. J Pharm Biomed Anal 4:377–387

Fitz-Patrick D, Patel YC (1981) Antibodies to insulin, pancreatic polypeptide, glucagon and somatostatin in insulin-treated diabetics. J Clin Endocrinol Metab 52:948–952

Forck G, Wilhelm E, Baumeister G, Westerloh K (1975) Scheinbare Insulinverträglichkeit bei einer Arthusreaktion durch Surfen. Med Welt 26:664–669

Forlani G, Santacroce G, Ciavarella A, Capelli M, Mattioli L, Vannini P (1986) Effects of mixing short- and intermediate-acting insulins on absorption course and biologic effect of short-acting preparation. Diabetes Care 9:587–590

Fort P (1981) Low-dose insulin infusion for diabetic ketoacidosis. Editorial correspondence. J Pediatr 98:169

Francis AJ, Hanning I, Alberti KGMM (1985) The effect of mixing human soluble and human crystalline zinc-suspension insulin: plasma insulin and blood glucose profiles after subcutaneous injection. Diabetic Medicine 2:177–180

Frank BH, Pekar AH, Veros AJ (1972) Insulin and proinsulin conformation in solution. Diabetes 21 (Suppl 2):486–491

Frank BH, Pettee JM, Zimmerman RE, Burck PJ (1981) The production of human proinsulin and its transformation to human insulin and C-peptide. In: Rich DH, Gross E (eds) Peptides: Synthesis-Structure-Function. Pierce Chemical Company, Rockford, pp 729–738

Fraser DT (1923) White mice and the assay of insulin. J Lab Clin Med 8:425–428

Fredericq E (1956) The association of insulin molecular units in aqueous solutions. Arch Biochem Biophys 65:218–228

Fredericq E, Neurath H (1950) The interaction of insulin with thiocyanate and other anions. The minimum molecular weight of insulin. J Am Chem Soc 72:2684–2691

Friesen H-J (1980) The relative reactivity of insulin amino groups as an indicator of structural accessibility and its use for synthetic approaches for structure-function studies. In: Brandenburg D, Wollmer A (eds) Insulin: Chemistry, structure and function of insulin and related hormones. Walter de Gruyter, Berlin New York, pp 125–133

Fullerton WW, Low BW (1970) Insulin crystallization in the presence of basic proteins and peptides. Biochim Biophys Acta 214:141–147

Furberg H, Jensen AK, Salbu B (1986) Effect of pretreatment with 0.9% sodium chloride or insulin solutions on the delivery of insulin from an infusion system. Am J Hosp Pharm 43:2209–2213

Galloway JA, Root MA (1972) New forms of insulin. Diabetes 21 (Suppl 2):637–648

Galloway JA, Root MA, Rathmacher RP, Carmichael RH (1973) A comparison of acid regular and neutral regular insulin. Responses of normal fasted subjects to varying doses of regular insulin. Diabetes 22:471–479

Galloway JA, Root MA, Chance RE, Jackson RL, Wentworth SM, Davidson JA (1975) New forms of insulin. In: Kryston LJ, Shaw RA (eds) Endocrinology and Diabetes, 30th Hahnemann Symposium. Grune & Stratton, New York, pp 329–342

Galloway JA, Kennedy ME, Marshall KA, Michael KR, Nimoy M, Raines KC, Spitzer TQ (1976) How to avoid clogging of insulin syringes. Diabetes Forecast 29, No.6 (Nov–Dec):27

Galloway JA, Spradlin CT, Root MA, Fineberg SE (1981 a) The plasma glucose response of normal fasting subjects to neutral regular and NPH biosynthetic human and purified pork insulins. Diabetes Care 4:183–188

Galloway JA, Spradlin CT, Nelson RL, Wentworth SM, Davidson JA, Swarner JL (1981 b) Factors influencing the absorption, serum insulin concentration, and blood glucose responses after injections of regular insulin and various insulin mixtures. Diabetes Care 4:366–376

Galloway JA, Spradlin CT, Jackson RL, Otto DC, Bechtel LD (1982) Mixtures of intermediate-acting insulin (NPH and Lente) with regular insulin: an update. In: Skyler JS (ed) Insulin Update, Excerpta Medica. Amsterdam Oxford Princeton, pp 111–119

Glauber HS, Revers RR, Henry R, Schmeiser L, Wallace P, Kolterman OG, Cohen RM, Rubenstein AH, Galloway JA, Frank BH, Olefsky JM (1986) In vivo deactivation of proinsulin action on glucose disposal and hepatic glucose production in normal man. Diabetes 35:311–317

Goeddel DV, Kleid DG, Bolivar F, Heyneker HL, Yansura DG, Crea R, Hirose T, Kraszewski A, Itakura K, Riggs AD (1979) Expression in Escherichia coli of chemically synthesized genes for human insulin. Proc Natl Acad Sci USA 76:106–110

Goerz G, Ruzicka T, Hofmann N, Drost H, Grüneklee D (1981) Granulomatöse allergische Reaktion vom verzögerten Typ auf Surfen. Hautarzt 32:187–190

Goldman J, Carpenter FH (1974) Zinc binding, circular dichroism, and equilibrium sedimentation studies on insulin (bovine) and several of its derivatives. Biochemistry 13:4566–4574

Goosen MFA, Leung YF, O'Shea GM, Chou S, Sun AM (1983) Long-acting insulin. Slow release of insulin from a biodegradable matrix implanted in diabetic rats. Diabetes 32:478–481

Gordon GS, Moses AC, Silver RD, Flier JS, Carey MC (1985) Nasal absorption of insulin: Enhancement by hydrophobic bile salts. Proc Natl Acad Sci USA 82:7419–7423

Graaff RAG de, Lewit-Bentley A, Tolley SP (1981) Effects of destabilizing agents on the insulin hexamer structure. In: Dodson G, Glusker J, Sayre D (eds) Structural studies on molecules of biological interest. Clarendon Press, Oxford, pp 547–556

Graham DT, Pomeroy AR (1978) The effects of freezing on commercial insulin suspensions. Int J Pharm 1:315–322

Graham DT, Pomeroy AR (1984) An in-vitro test for the duration of action of insulin suspensions. J Pharm Pharmacol 36:427–430

Grant PT, Coombs TL, Frank BH (1972) Differences in the nature of the interaction of insulin and proinsulin with zinc. Biochem J 126:433–440

Grau U (1985) Chemical stability of insulin in a delivery system environment. Diabetologia 28:458–463

Grau U, Seipke G, Obermeier R, Thurow H (1982) Stabile Insulinlösungen für automatische Dosiergeräte. In: Petersen K-G, Schlüter KJ, Kerp L (Hrsg) Neue Insuline. Freiburg Graphische Betriebe, Freiburg, pp 411–418

Hagedorn HC (1946) The absorption of protamine insulin. Rep Steno Hosp (Cph) 1:25–28

Hagedorn HC, Jensen BN, Krarup NB, Wodstrup I (1936) Protamine insulinate. J Am Med Assoc 106:177–180

Haines BA Jr., Martin AN (1961) Interfacial properties of powdered material; caking in liquid dispersions I. Caking and flocculation studies. J Pharm Sci 50:228–232

Hallas-Møller K (1945) Chemical and biological insulin studies I and II. Dissertation. Copenhagen University

Hallas-Møller K (1956) The Lente insulins. Diabetes 5:7–14

Hallas-Møller K, Petersen K, Schlichtkrull J (1951) Crystalline and amorphous insulin-zinc compounds with prolonged action (in Danish). Ugeskr Laeger 113:1761–1767

Hallas-Møller K, Petersen K, Schlichtkrull J (1952) Crystalline and amorphous insulin-zinc compounds with prolonged action. Science 116:394–399

Harding MM, Hodgkin DC, Kennedy AF, O'Connor A, Weitzmann PDJ (1966) The crystal structure of insulin. II. An investigation of rhombohedral zinc insulin crystals and a report of other crystalline forms. J Mol Biol 16:212–226

Harfenist EJ, Craig LC (1952) Countercurrent distribution studies with insulin. J Am Chem Soc 74:3083–3087

Havlová M, Nobilis M, Patočka L (1969) Stability of Superdep insulin (in Czechoslovakian). Cesk Farm 18:390–392

Heding LG (1971) Radioimmunological determination of pancreatic and gut glucagon in plasma. Diabetologia 7:10–19

Heding LG, Larsen UD, Markussen J, Jørgensen KH, Hallund O (1974) Radioimmunoassays for human, pork and ox C-peptides and related substances. In: Levine R, Pfeiffer EF (eds) Radioimmunoassay: Methodology and applications in physiology and in clinical studies. Georg Thieme Publishers, Stuttgart, pp 40–44

Heding LG, Larsson Y, Ludvigsson J (1980) The immunogenicity of insulin preparation. Antibody levels before and after transfer to highly purified porcine insulin. Diabetologia 19:511–515

Heding LG, Marshall MO, Persson B, Dahlquist G, Thalme B, Lindgren F, Åkerblom HK, Rilva A, Knip M, Ludvigsson J, Stenhammar L, Strömberg L, Søvik O, Bævre H, Wefring K, Vidnes J, Kjærgård JJ, Bro P, Kaad PH (1984) Immunogenicity of monocomponent human and porcine insulin in newly diagnosed type 1 (insulin-dependent) diabetic children. Diabetologia 27:96–98

Hefford MA, Oda G, Kaplan H (1986) Structure-function relationships in the free insulin monomer. Biochem J 237:663–668

Heine RJ, Bilo HJG, Fonk T, Veen EA van der, Meer J van der (1984) Adsorption kinetics and action profiles of mixtures of short- and intermediate-acting insulins. Diabetologia 27:558–562

Helbig H-J (1976) Insulindimere aus der b-Komponente von Insulinpräparationen. Rheinisch-Westfälische Technische Hochschule, Aachen (Dissertation)

Hemmingsen AM, Krogh A (1926) The assay of insulin by the convulsive-dose method on white mice. League of Nations Health III. 7:40–46

Hildebrandt P, Birch K, Sestoft L, Vølund Aa (1984) Dose-dependent subcutaneous absorption of porcine, bovine and human NPH insulins. Acta Med Scand 215:69–73

Hildebrandt P, Berger A, Vølund Aa, Kühl C (1985) The subcutaneous absorption of human and bovine ultralente insulin formulations. Diabetic Medicine 2:355–359

Hildebrandt R, Ilius A, Lotz U, Schliack V (1984) Effect of insulin suppositories in type I diabetic patients (preliminary communication). Exp Clin Endocrinol 83:168–172

Hirai S, Ikenaga T, Matsuzawa T (1978) Nasal absorption of insulin in dogs. Diabetes 27:296–299

Hirai S, Yashiki T, Mima H (1981) Effect of surfactants on the nasal absorption of insulin in rats. Int J Pharm 9:165–172

Hirata Y, Kohama T, Ooi K (1983) Nasal administration of insulin in healthy subjects and diabetic patients. In: Sakamoto N, Alberti KGMM (eds) Current and future therapies with insulin. Excerpta Medica, Amsterdam Oxford Princeton, pp 263–267

Hirn S, Königstein RP, Pietschmann H (1982) Langzeitanwendung von Des-Phe-Insulin. In: Petersen K-G, Schlüter KJ, Kerp L (Hrsg) Neue Insuline. Freiburger Graphische Betriebe, Freiburg, pp 384–389

Hirsch JI, Wood JH, Thomas RB (1981) Insulin adsorption to polyolefin infusion bottles and polyvinyl chloride administration sets. Am J Hosp Pharm 38:995–997

Hodgkin DC (1974) Varieties of insulin. J Endocrinol 63:3P–14P

Hoffmann R, Rühl J (1982) Insulinverluste an Infusionsmaterial. Medizinische Fakultät der Universität Düsseldorf (Dissertation)

Holladay LA, Ascoli M, Puett D (1977) Conformational stability and self-association of zinc-free bovine insulin at neutral pH. Biochim Biophys Acta 494:245–254

Holman RR, Steemson J, Darling P, Reeves WG, Turner RC (1984) Human ultralente insulin. Br Med J 288:665–668

Home PD, Mann NP, Hutchison AS, Park R, Walford S, Murphy M, Reeves WG (1984) A fifteen-month double-blind cross-over study of the efficacy and antigenicity of human and pork insulins. Diabetic Medicine 1:93–98

Horrow JC (1985) Protamine: a review of its toxicity. Anesth Analg 64:348–361

Howell SL, Tyhurst M, Duvefelt H, Andersson A, Hellerström C (1978) Role of zinc and calcium in the formation and storage of insulin in the pancreatic B-cell. Cell Tissue Res 188:107–118

Humbel RE, Bosshard HR, Zahn H (1972) Chemistry of insulin. In: Greep RO, Astwood EB (eds) Endocrinology. Handbook of Physiology, section 7, vol I,. American Physiological Society, Washington DC, pp 111–132

Ichikawa K, Ohata I, Mitomi M, Kawamura S, Maeno H, Kawata H (1980) Rectal absorption of insulin suppositories in rabbits. J Pharm Pharmacol 32:314–318

Irsigler K, Kritz H (1979) Long-term continuous intravenous insulin therapy with a portable insulin dosage-regulating apparatus. Diabetes 28:196–203

Irsigler K, Kritz H, Hagmüller G, Franetzki M, Prestele K, Thurow H, Geisen K (1981) Long-term continuous intraperitoneal insulin infusion with an implanted remote-controlled insulin infusion device. Diabetes 30:1072–1075

Ishida M, Machida Y, Nambu N, Nagai T (1981) New mucosal dosage form of insulin. Chem Pharm Bull (Tokyo) 29:810–816

Jackman WS, Lougheed W, Marliss EB, Zinman B, Albisser AM (1980) For insulin infusion: A miniature precision peristaltic pump and silicone rubber reservoir. Diabetes Care 3:322–331

Jackson RL, Storvick WO, Hollinden CS, Stroeh LE, Stilz JG (1972) Neutral regular insulin. Diabetes 21:235–245

Jackson RL, Bilginturan N, Murthy DYN, England J (1977) New improved insulins. In: Laron Z (ed) Pediatric adolescent endocrinology, vol 2. F. Karger, Basel, pp 105–109

James DE, Jenkins AB, Kraegen EW, Chisholm DJ (1981) Insulin precipitation in artificial infusion devices. Diabetologia 21:554–557

Jaques LB (1949) A study of the toxicity of the protamine, salmine. Br J Pharmacol 4:135–144

Jefferson IG, Marteau TM, Smith MA, Baum JD (1985) A multiple injection regimen using an insulin injection pen and pre-filled cartridged soluble human insulin in adolescents with diabetes. Diabetic Medicine 2:493–497

Jeffrey PD (1974) Polymerization behaviour of bovine zinc-insulin at neutral pH. Molecular weight of the subunit and the effect of glucose. Biochemistry 13:4441–4447

Jeffrey PD, Coates JH (1966a) An equilibrium ultracentrifuge study of the self-association of bovine insulin. Biochemistry 5:489–498

Jeffrey PD, Coates JH (1966b) An equilibrium ultracentrifuge study of the effect of ionic strength on the self-association of bovine insulin. Biochemistry 5:3820–3824

Jeffrey PD, Milthorpe BK, Nichol LW (1976) Polymerization pattern of insulin at pH 7.0. Biochemistry 15:4660–4665

Jensen HF (1938) Administration of insulin. In: Insulin. Its chemistry and physiology. Commonwealth Foundation, New York, pp 92–111

Jørgensen KH, Brange J, Hallund O, Pingel M (1970) A method for the preparation of essentially pure insulin. In: Rodrigues RR, Ebling FJG, Henderson I, Assan R (eds) Seventh Congress of the International Diabetes Federation. Excerpta Medica Foundation, Amsterdam New York London Milan Tokyo Buenos Aires (International Congress Series No. 209, Abstracts, p 149)

Jørgensen KH, Hallund O, Heding LG, Tronier B, Falholt K, Damgaard U, Thim L, Brange J (1982) Estimation of insulin purity in light of developments in analytical methods. In: Gueriguian JL, Bransome ED, Outschoorn AS (eds) Hormone Drugs. United States Pharmacopeial Convention, Rockville, Maryland, pp 139–147

Jorpes JE (1949) Recrystallized insulin for diabetic patients with insulin allergy. Arch Intern Med 83:363–371

Kaplan H, Hefford MA, Chan AM-L, Oda G (1984) Chemical reactivity of the functional groups of insulin. Concentration-dependence studies. Biochem J 217:135–143

Kasama T, Iwata Y, Okubo T, Sakaguchi Y, Sugiura M (1980) Determination of purity and identification of animal sources of insulin in various insulin preparations. Jpn J Pharmacol 30:293–300

Kasama T, Iwata Y, Oshiro K, Uchida M, Sakaguchi Y, Namie K, Sugiura M (1981) Antigenicity of desamido-insulin and monocomponent insulin. Diabetologia 21:65–69

Kerchner J, Colaluca DM, Juhl RP (1980) Effect of whole blood on insulin adsorption onto intravenous infusion systems. Am Jm Hosp Pharm 37:1323–1325

Kern RA, Langner PH (1939) Protamine and allergy. J Am Med Assoc 113:198–200

Kerp L, Steinhilber S, Kasemir H, Han J, Henrichs HR, Geiger R (1974) Changes in immunospecificity and biologic activity of bovine insulin due to subsequent removal of the amino acids B_1, B_2 and B_3. Diabetes 23:651–656

Klostermeyer H, Zahn H (1971) Struktur, Eigenschaften und Synthese des Insulins. In: Dörzbach E (Hrsg) Insulin. Handbuch der experimentellen Pharmakologie, Bd XXXII/1. Springer, Berlin Heidelberg New York, pp 273–312

Knape JTA, Schuller JL, de Haan P, de Jong AP, Bovill JG (1981) An anaphylactic reaction to protamine in a patient allergic to fish. Anesthesiology 55:324–325

Kraegen EW, Lazarus L, Meler H, Campbell L, Chia YO (1975) Carrier solutions for low-level intravenous insulin infusion. Br Med J 3:464–466

Krause U, Beyer J (1975) Die Reinheit handelsüblicher Insulinzubereitungen. Dtsch Med Wochenschr 100:238–240

Krayenbühl C, Poulsen JE (1959) Protamine-zinc-insulin in crystalline suspension. Dan Med Bull 6:270–272

Krayenbühl C, Rosenberg T (1946) Crystalline protamine insulin. Rep Steno Mem Hosp Nord Insulinlab 1:60–73

Kroeff EP, Chance RE (1982) Applications of high performance liquid chromatography for the analysis of insulins. In: Gueriguian JL, Bransome ED, Outschoorn AS (eds) Hormone Drugs. United States Pharmacopeial Convention, Rockville, Maryland, pp 148–162

Krogh A, Hemmingsen AM (1928) The destructive action of heat on insulin solutions. Biochem J 22:1231–1238

Kruse V, Heding LG, Jørgensen KH, Tronier B, Christensen M, Thim L, Frank BH, Root MA, Cohen RM, Rubenstein AH (1984) Human proinsulin standards. Diabetologia 27:414–415

Kulpe W (1958) Hautnekrosen bei der Insulinbehandlung durch Surfen-Überempfindlichkeit. Muench Med Wochenschr 100:998–999

Kumar D (1979) Immunoreactivity of insulin antibodies in insulin-treated diabetics. Significance of the beta-chain carboxyterminal amino acid (B-30) of insulin. Diabetes 28:994–1000

Kumar D, Miller LV (1970) Pork insulin resistance treated with dealaninated insulin. Diabetes (Suppl) 19:392 (abstract)

Kurtz AB, Gray RS, Markanday S, Nabarro JDN (1983) Circulating IgG antibody to protamine in patients treated with protamine-insulins. Diabetologia 25:322–324

Lacey AH (1967) The unit of insulin. Diabetes 16:198–200

Lange RH, Blödorn J, Magdowski G, Trampisch HJ (1979) Crystalline preparations of rhombohedral porcine insulin as studied by electron diffraction. J Ultrastruct Res 68:81–91

Langkjær L, Brange J (1982) Preloading of insulin syringes. Diabetologia 23:182–183 (abstract)

Lauritzen T, Pramming S (1984) Insulin pumps – still a research tool? Ann Clin Res 16:98–106

Lauritzen T, Deckert T, Frost-Larsen K, Svendsen PAa, Larsen H-W, Christiansen JS, Parving H-H, Binder C, Nerup J, Deckert M, Larsen A, Lørup B, Bojsen J, Beck-Jansen L (1982) One year's experience of insulin pumps in diabetes. Nord Med 97:130–133

Lauritzen T, Thorsteinsson B, Pramming S, Sørensen L, Binder C (1984) Subcutaneous absorption of U-40 and U-100 insulin. Horm Metabol Res 16:611–612

Lautenschläger KL, Dörzbach E, Schaumann O (1937) Verfahren zur Herstellung von Präparaten aus dem blutzuckersenkenden Hormon der Bauchspeicheldrüse. D R Patent 727888

Lens J (1947) The inactivation of insulin solutions. J Biol Chem 169:313–322

Levandoski LA, White NH, Santiago JV (1982) Localized skin reactions to insulin: Insulin lipodystrophies and skin reactions to pumped subcutaneous insulin therapy. Diabetes Care 5:6–10

Li CH (1954) Protein hormones. In: Neurath H, Bailey K (eds) The proteins, vol II/A. Acad Press, New York, p 636

Ling V, Jergil B, Dixon GH (1971) The biosynthesis of protamine in trout testis. III. Characterization of protamine components and their synthesis during testis development. J Biol Chem 246:1168–1176

Little JA, Arnott JH (1966) Sulfated insulin in mild, moderate, severe, and insulin-resistant diabetes mellitus. Diabetes 15:457–465

Little JA, Lee R, Sebriakova M, Csima A (1977) Insulin antibodies and clinical complications in diabetics treated for five years with Lente or sulfated insulin. Diabetes 26:980–988

Liversidge GG, Nishihata T, Engle KK, Higuchi T (1985) Effect of rectal suppository formulation on the release of insulin and on the glucose plasma levels in dogs. Int J Pharm 23:87–95

Lloyd LF (1982) Analysis of insulin preparations by high-performance liquid chromatography. Anal Proc (London) 19:131–133

Lloyd LF, Corran PH (1982) Analysis of insulin preparations by reversed-phase high-performance liquid chromatography. J Chromatogr 240:445–454

Lougheed WD, Woulfe-Flanagan H, Clement JR, Albisser AM (1980) Insulin aggregation in artifical delivery systems. Diabetologia 19:1–9

Lougheed WD, Albisser AM, Martindale HM, Chow JC, Clement JR (1983) Physical stability of insulin formulations. Diabetes 32:424–432

Low BW (1952) Orientation of the polypeptide chains in crystals of acid insulin sulphate. Nature 169:955–956

Low BW, Chen CCH (1969) Monoclinic insulin crystals. J Mol Biol 43:227–229

Ludvigsson J (1984) Insulin antibodies in diabetic children treated with monocomponent porcine insulin from the onset: relationship to B-cell function and partial remission. Diabetologia 26:138–141

Luyckx AS, Daubresse J-C, Jaminet C, Scheen A, Lefebvre PJ (1986) Immunogenicity of semi-synthetic human insulin in man. Long-term comparison with porcine monocomponent insulin. Acta Diabetol Lat 23:101–106

Maislos M, Mead PM, Gaynor DH, Robbins DC (1986) The source of the circulating aggregate of insulin in type I diabetic patients is therapeutic insulin. J Clin Invest 77:717–723

Marcker K (1960) The binding of the "structural" zinc ions in crystalline insulin. Acta Chem Scand 14:2071–2074

Marks HP (1925) The biological assay of insulin preparations in comparison with a stable standard. Br Med J II:1102–1104

Markussen J (1980) US Patent 4343898

Markussen J (1982) Human Monocomponent aus Schweine-Rohinsulin. In: Petersen K-G, Schlüter KJ, Kerp L (Hrsg) Neue Insuline. Freiburger Graphische Betriebe, Freiburg, pp 38–44

Markussen J, Schaumburg K (1983) Reaction mechanism in trypsin catalyzed synthesis of human insulin studied by ^{17}O-NMR spectroscopy. In: Peptides 1982. Blaha K, Malon P (eds) Proceedings 17th European Peptide Symposium, Prague. Walter de Gruyter, Berlin New York, pp 387–394

Markussen J, Jørgensen KH, Heding LG (1970) Preparation of bovine ^{125}I-tyrosyl-C-peptide. Horm Metab Res 2:53–55

Markussen J, Damgaard U, Jørgensen KH, Rasmussen E, Snel L, Thim L, Voigt HO (1982) Production of human monocomponent insulin. In: Gueriguian JL, Bransome ED, Outschoorn AS (eds) Hormone Drugs. United States Pharmacopeial Convention, Rockville, Maryland, pp 116–126

Markussen J, Damgaard U, Diers I, Fiil N, Hansen MT, Larsen P, Norris F, Norris K, Schou O, Snel L, Thim L, Voigt HO (1986a) Biosynthesis of human insulin in yeast via single chain precursors. Diabetologia 29:568A–569A (abstract)

Markussen J, Damgaard U, Diers I, Fiil N, Hansen MT, Larsen P, Norris F, Norris K, Schou O, Snel L, Thim L, Voigt HO (1986b) Biosynthesis of human insulin in yeast via single-chain precursors. In: Theodoropoulos (ed) Peptides. 1986: Walter de Gruyter, Berlin (in press)

Marliss EB (1982) Insulin: Sixty years of use. N Engl J Med 306:362–364

Melberg SG, Havelund S, Villumsen, J, Brange J (1987) Insulin compatibility with polymer materials used in external pump infusion systems. Diabetic Medicine. Submitted for publication

Menczel J, Levy M, Bentwich Z (1966) Insulin resistant diabetes treated with sulphated insulin. Isr J Med Sci 2:764–768

Miles AA, Mussett MV, Perry WLM (1952) Third international standard for insulin. Bull WHO 7:445–459

Milthorpe BK, Nichol LW, Jeffrey PD (1977) The polymerization pattern of zinc(II)-insulin at pH 7.0. Biochim Biophys Acta 495:195–202

Mirsky IA, Kawamura K (1966) Heterogeneity of crystalline insulin. Endocrinology 78:1115–1119

Mitrano FP, Newton DW (1982) Factors affecting insulin adherence to type I glass bottles. Am J Hosp Pharm 39:1491–1495

Mizuno N, Ogawa T, Ishida M, Okada K, Shigeaki B (1980) Pancreatic polypeptide binding antibodies in insulin-treated diabetics. J Jpn Diabetic Soc 23:219–226

Moloney PJ, Aprile MA, Wilson S (1964) Sulfated insulin for treatment of insulin-resistant diabetics. J New Drugs 4:258–263

Moorthy SS, Pond W, Rowland RG (1980) Severe circulatory shock following protamine (an anaphylactic reaction). Anesth Analg 59:77–78

Moses AC, Gordon GS, Carey MC, Flier JS (1983) Insulin administered intranasally as an insulin-bile salt aerosol. Effectiveness and reproducibility in normal and diabetic subjects. Diabetes 32:1040–1047

Nathan DM, Axelrod L, Flier JS, Carr DB (1981) U-500 insulin in the treatment of antibody-mediated insulin resistance. Ann Int Med 94:653–656

Neubauer HP, Obermeier R, Schnorr G (1984) Immunological properties and biological effectiveness of insulin analogues substituted at position B30. Diabetologia 27:129–131

Nishihata T, Rytting JH, Kamada A, Higuchi T, Routh M, Caldwell L (1983) Enhancement of rectal absorption of insulin using salicylates in dogs. J Pharm Pharmacol 35:148–151

Nishihata T, Okamura Y, Kamada A, Higuchi T, Yagi T, Kawamori R, Shichiri M (1985) Enhanced bioavailability of insulin after rectal administration with enamine as adjuvant in depancreatized dogs. J Pharm Pharmacol 37:22–26

Nolte MS, Poon V, Grodsky GM, Forsham PH, Karam JH (1983) Reduced solubility of short-acting soluble insulins when mixed with longer-acting insulins. Diabetes 32:1177–1181

Nordström L, Fletcher R, Pavek K (1978) Shock of anaphylactoid type induced by protamine: a continuous cardiorespiratory record. Acta Anaesthesiol Scand 22:195–201

Oberly K, Clark JL, Paulshock BZ (1979) Sterility of insulin stored in syringes. Diabetes Care 2:531

Ohta M, Tokunaga H, Kimura T, Satoh H, Kawamura J (1983) Analysis of insulins by high-performance liquid chromatography. II. Separation of various species of insulins. Chem Pharm Bull (Tokyo) 31:3566–3570

O'Neill JJ, Mead CA (1982) The parabens: Bacterial adaptation and preservative capacity. J Soc Cosmet Chem 33:75–84

Oppenheim RC, Stewart NF, Gordon L, Patel HM (1982) The production and evaluation of orally administered insulin nanoparticles. Drug Dev Ind Pharm 8:531–546

Ornstein L (1964) Disc electrophoresis-I. Ann NY Acad Sci 121:321–349

Orr NA, Spence J (1977) Applications of particle size analysis in the pharmaceutical industry. Analyst 102:466–472

Owens DR (1986) Human insulin: Clinical pharmacological studies in normal man. MTP Press Limited, Lancaster Boston The Hague Dordrecht. Thesis

Owens DR, Jones MK, Hayes TM, Heding LG, Alberti KGMM, Home PD, Burrin JM, Newcombe RG (1981) Human insulin: study of safety and efficacy in man. Br Med J 282:1264–1266

Owens DR, Jones IR, Birtwell AJ, Burge CTR, Luzio S, Davies CJ, Heyburn P, Heding LG (1984) Study of porcine and human isophane (NPH) insulins in normal subjects. Diabetologia 26:261–265

Owens DR, Vora JP, Heding LG, Luzio S, Ryder REJ, Atiea J, Hayes TM (1986) Human, porcine and bovine ultralente insulin: Subcutaneous administration in normal man. Diabetic Medicine 3:326–329

Patel YC, Reichlin S (1979) Somatostatin. In: Jaffe BM, Behrman HR (eds) Methods of hormone radioimmunoassay. Academic Press, New York, pp 77–99

Pekar AH, Frank BH (1972) Conformation of proinsulin. A comparison of insulin and proinsulin self-association at neutral pH. Biochemistry 11:4013–4016

Petersen K (1945) Method of producing crystalline insulin. US Patent 2626228

Pfeiffer EF, Thum C, Clemens AH (1974) The artificial β-cell – a continuous control of blood sugar by external regulation of insulin infusion (glucose controlled insulin infusion system). Horm Metab Res 6:339–342

Phillips M, Simpson RW, Holman RR, Turner RC (1979) A simple and rational twice daily insulin regime. Q J Med New series 48:493–506

Pickup JC, Keen H, Viberti GC, White MC, Kohner EM, Parsons JA, Alberti KGMM (1980) Continuous subcutaneous insulin infusion in the treatment of diabetes mellitus. Diabetes Care 2:290–300

Pietri A, Raskin P (1981) Cutaneous complications of chronic continuous subcutaneous insulin infusion therapy. Diabetes Care 4:624–626

Pingel M, Vølund Aa (1972) Stability of insulin preparations. Diabetes 21:805–813

Pingel M, Vølund Aa, Sørensen E, Sørensen AR (1982) Assessment of insulin potency by chemical and biological methods. In: Gueriguian JL, Bransome ED, Outschoorn AS (eds) Hormone Drugs. United States Pharmacopeial Convention. Rockville, Maryland, pp 200–207

Pingel M, Vølund Aa, Sørensen E, Collins JE, Dieter CT (1985) Biological potency of porcine, bovine and human insulins in the rabbit bioassay system. Diabetologia 28:862–869

Pitts JE, Wood SP, Horuk R, Bedarkar S, Blundell TL (1980) Pancreatic hormone storage granules: The role of metal ions and polypeptide oligomers. In: Brandenburg D, Wollmer A (eds) Insulin. Chemistry, structure and function of insulin and related hormones. Walther de Gruyter, Berlin New York, pp 673–682

Pocker Y, Biswas SB (1980) Conformational dynamics of insulin in solution. Circular dichroic studies. Biochemistry 19:5043–5049

Pocker Y, Biswas SB (1981) Self-association of insulin and the role of hydrophobic bonding: A thermodynamic model of insulin dimerization. Biochemistry 20:4354–4361

Pongor S, Brownlee M, Cerami A (1983) Preparation of high-potency, non-aggregating insulins using a novel sulfation procedure. Diabetes 32:1087–1091

Pontiroli AE, Alberetto M, Secchi A, Dossi G, Bosi I, Pozza G (1982) Insulin given intranasally induces hypoglycaemia in normal and diabetic subjects. Brit Med J 284:303–306

Poulsen JE, Deckert T (1976) Insulin preparations and the clinical us of insulin. Acta Med Scand (Suppl) 601:197–245

Prestele K, Franetzki M, Kresse H (1980) Development of program-controlled portable insulin delivery devices. Diabetes Care 3:362–368

Pullen RA, Lindsay DG, Wood SP, Tickle IJ, Blundell TL, Wollmer A, Krail G, Brandenburg D, Zahn H, Gliemann J, Gammeltoft S (1976) Receptor-binding region of insulin. Nature 259:369–373

Purintun LR, McGrane HF (1972) A survey of sterilization procedures recommended to diabetic patients. Health Serv Rep 87:357–364

Ramesh V, Bradbury JH (1986) ^{1}H NMR studies of insulin. Reversible transformation of 2-zinc to 4-zinc insulin hexamer. Int J Pept Protein Res 28:146–153

Rasch R (1979) Control of blood glucose levels in the streptozotocin diabetic rat using a long-acting heat-treated insulin. Diabetologia 16:185–190

Reiner L, Searle DS, Lang EH (1939) On the hypoglycemic activity of globin insulin. J Pharmacol Exp Ther 67:330–340

Renneboog-Squilbin C, Delhaise P, Wodak S (1981) The influence of crystal packing on the 3-dimensional conformation of insulin. Arch Int Physiol Biochim 89:B192–B193

Revers RR, Henry R, Schmeiser L, Kolterman O, Cohen R, Rubenstein A, Frank B, Galloway J, Olefsky JM (1984) Biosynthetic human insulin and proinsulin have additive but not synergistic effects on total body glucose disposal. J Clin Endocrinol Metab 58:1094–1098

Ritschel WA, Ritschel GB (1984) Rectal administration of insulin. Methods Find Exp Clin Pharmacol 6:513–529

Rivier J, McClintock R (1983) Reversed-phase high-performance liquid chromatography of insulins from different species. J Chromatogr 268:112–119

Robbins DC, Shoelson SE, Tager HS, Mead PM, Gaynor DH (1985) Products of therapeutic insulins in the blood of insulin-dependent (type I) diabetic patients. Diabetes 34:510–519

Rolando RL, Torroba D (1972) Heterogeneity of the fourth international standard for insulin by gel-chromatography on Sephadex. Experientia 28:1169

Romans RG, Scott DA, Fisher AM (1940) Preparation of crystalline insulin. Ind Eng Chem 32:908–910

Rosenbloom AL (1974) Advances in commercial insulin preparations. Am J Dis Child 128:631–633

Rosenbloom AL, Londono JH, Jordan J, Rosenbloom EK (1971) U 100 insulin: Trial of Lente and Regular in 50 children with diabetes. Physicians Drug Man 2:142–144

Rowles B, Sperandio GJ, Shaw SM (1971) Effects of elastomer closures on the sorption of certain ^{14}C-labelled drug and preservative combinations. Bull Parenteral Drug Assoc 25:2–22

Sachse G, Federlin K (1981) Sind Des-Phe-Insulin-haltige Insulinmischungen handelsüblichen Präparaten vorzuziehen? Med Klin 76:319–323

Sachse G, Mäser E, Federlin K (1982) Kurz- und Langzeittherapie mit Des-Phe-insulinhaltigen Insulinen. In: Petersen KG, Schlüter KJ, Kerp L (Hrsg) Neue Insuline. Freiburger Graphische Betriebe, Freiburg, pp 317–324

Saffran M, Kumar GS, Savariar C, Burnham JC, Williams F, Neckers DC (1986) A new approach to the oral administration of insulin and other peptide drugs. Science 233:1081–1084

Sahyun M, Nixon A, Goodell M (1939) Influence of certain metals on the stability of insulin. J Pharmacol Exp Ther 65:143–149

Salzman R, Manson JE, Griffing GT, Kimmerle R, Ruderman N, McCall A, Stoltz EI. Mullin C, Small D, Armstrong J, Melby JC (1985) Intranasal aerosolized insulin. Mixed-meal studies and long-term use in type I diabetes. N Engl J Med 312:1078–1084

Samuel T (1977) Antibodies reacting with salmon and human protamines in sera from infertile men and from vasectomized men and monkeys. Clin Exp Immunol 30:181–187

Samuel T, Kolk AHJ, Rümke P (1978) Studies on the immunogenicity of protamines in humans and experimental animals by means of a micro-complement fixation test. Clin Exp Immunol 33:252–260

Sanchez MB, Paolillo M, Chacon RS, Camejo M (1982) Protamine as a cause of generalised allergic reactions to NPH insulin. Lancet I:1243

Sanger F (1959) Chemistry of insulin. Science 129:1340–1344

Sanger F, Thompson EOP, Kitai R (1955) The amide groups of insulin. Biochem J 59:509–518

Santeusanio F, Massi-Benedetti M, Clementi A, Calabrese G, Bueti A, Picchio E, Brunetti P (1981) Clinical trial with porcine Des-Phe^{B1} insulin. A comparative study with unmodified insulin on therapeutical efficacy, biological activity and immunogenicity. Diabete Metab 7:173–179

Sato S, Jeong SY, McRea JC, Kim SW (1984) Self-regulating insulin delivery systems. II. In vitro studies. J Controlled Release 1:67–77

Schade DS, Eaton RP (1982) Bactericidal properties of commercial USP formulated insulin. Diabetes 31:36–39

Schade DS, Eaton RP, Spencer W (1981) Implantation of an artificial pancreas. Current perspectives. J Am Med Assoc 245:709–710

Schade DS, Eaton RP, Edwards WS, Doberneck RC, Spencer WJ, Carlson GA, Bair RE, Love JT, Urenda RS, Gaona JI (1982a) A remotely programmable insulin delivery system. Successful short-term implantation in man. J Amer Med Assoc 247:1848–1853

Schade DS, Eaton RP, DeLongo J, Saland LC, Ladman AJ, Carlson GA (1982b) Electron microscopy of insulin precipitates. Diabetes Care 5:25–30

Scheller JC, Galloway JA (1975) The development of the insulin unit. Am J Pharm 147:29–32

Schernthaner G, Borkenstein M, Fink M, Mayr WR, Menzel J, Schober E (1983) Immunogenicity of human monocomponent or pork monocomponent insulin in HLA-DR-typed insulin-dependent diabetic individuals. Diabetes Care 6:43–48

Schernthaner G, Schober E, Borkenstein M (1984) Insulin-antibody-free state in human-insulin treated type-I diabetics is associated with increased endogenous insulin production. Diabetes 33, Suppl 1:12A (abstract)

Schildt B, Ahlgren T, Berghem L, Wendet Y (1978) Adsorption of insulin by infusion materials. Acta Anaesthesiol Scand 22:556–562

Schlichtkrull J (1956a) Insulin crystals I. The minimum mole-fraction of metal in infusion crystals prepared with Zn^{++}, Cd^{++}, Co^{++}, Ni^{++}, Cu^{++}, Mn^{++}, or Fe^{++}. Acta Chem Scand 10:1455–1458

Schlichtkrull J (1956b) Insulin crystals II. Shape of rhombohedral zinc-insulin crystals in relation to species and crystallization media. Acta Chem Scand 10:1459–1464

Schlichtkrull J (1957a) Insulin Crystals III. Determination of the rhombehedral zinc-insulin unit-cell by combined microscopical and chemical examinations. Acta Chem Scand 11:291–298

Schlichtkrull J (1957b) Insulin Crystals IV. The Preparation of nuclei, seeds and monodisperse insulin crystal suspensions. Acta Chem Scand 11:299–302

Schlichtkrull J (1957c) Insulin Crystals V. The nucleation and growth of insulin crystals. Acta Chem Scand 11:439–460

Schlichtkrull J (1957d) Insulin Crystals VI. The anisotropic growth of insulin crystals. Acta Chem Scand 11:484–486

Schlichtkrull J (1957e) Insulin Crystals VII. The growth of insulin crystals. Acta Chem Scand 11:1248–1256

Schlichtkrull J (1958) Insulin crystals. Chemical and biological studies on insulin crystals and insulin zinc suspensions. Thesis, first edn. Ejnar Munksgaard Publisher, Copenhagen

Schlichtkrull J (1959) New insulin crystal suspensions with various timings of action and contain-
    ing no added zinc. In: Oberdisse K, Jahnke K (eds) Diabetes Mellitus III. Kongress der In-
    ternational Diabetes Federation Düsseldorf. 21–25. Juni 1958, Georg Thieme, Stuttgart,
    pp 773–777
Schlichtkrull J (1974) Antigenicity of monocomponent insulins. Lancet II:1260–1261
Schlichtkrull J (1977a) Purity and antigenicity of insulin preparations. Acta Paediatr Scand
    [Suppl] 270:37–40
Schlichtkrull J (1977b) The absorption of insulin. Acta Paediatr Scand [Suppl] 270:97–102
Schlichtkrull J, Funder J, Munck O (1961) Clinical evaluation of a new insulin preparation. In:
    Demole M (ed) 4e Congrès de la Féderation internationale du Diabète, Genève. Editions
    Médecine et Hygiène, Genève, I: pp 303–305
Schlichtkrull J, Munck O, Jersild M (1965) Insulin Rapitard and Insulin Actrapid. Acta Med
    Scand 177:103–113
Schlichtkrull J, Brange J, Ege H, Hallund O, Heding LG, Jørgensen K, Markussen J, Stahnke
    P, Sundby F, Vølund Aa (1970) Proinsulin and related proteins. Diabetologia 6:80–81
    (abstract)
Schlichtkrull J, Brange J, Christiansen AaH, Hallund O, Heding LG, Jørgensen KH (1972) Clini-
    cal aspects of insulin – antigenicity. Diabetes 21 (Suppl 2):649–656
Schlichtkrull J, Brange J, Christiansen AaH, Hallund O, Heding LG, Jørgensen KH, Rasmussen
    SM, Sørensen E, Vølund Aa (1974) Monocomponent insulin and its clinical implications.
    Horm Metab Res (Suppl Ser) 5:134–143
Schlichtkrull J, Pingel M, Heding LG, Brange J, Jørgensen KH (1975a) Insulin preparations
    with prolonged effect. In: Hasselblatt A, Bruchhausen F von (eds) Handbook of Experimen-
    tal Pharmacology, New Series, vol XXXII/2, Springer-Verlag, Berlin Heidelberg New York,
    pp 729–777
Schlichtkrull J, Ege H, Jørgensen KH, Markussen J, Sundby F (1975b) Die Chemie des Insulins.
    In: Oberdisse K (Hrsg) Diabetes mellitus A (Handbuch der Inneren Medizin, Bd 7/2A).
    Springer, Berlin Heidelberg New York, pp 77–127
Schmidt DD, Arens A (1968) Proinsulin vom Rind. Isolierung, Eigenschaften und seine Aktivie-
    rung durch Trypsin. Hoppe-Seyler's Z Physiol Chem 349:1157–1168
Scott DA (1934) Crystalline insulin. Biochem J 28:1592–1602
Scott DA, Fisher AM (1936) Studies on insulin with protamine. J Pharmacol Exp Ther 58:78–
    92
Sefton MV, Antonacci GM (1984) Adsorption isotherms of insulin onto various materials. Di-
    abetes 33:674–680
Sestoft L, Vølund Aa, Gammeltoft S, Birch K, Hildebrandt P (1982) The biological properties
    of human insulin. Subcutaneous absorption, receptor binding and the clinical effect in dia-
    betics assessed by a new statistical method. Acta Med Scand 212:21–28
Sheffer MG, Kaplan H (1979) Unusual chemical properties of the amino groups of insulin: im-
    plications for structure-function relationship. Can J Biochem 57:489–496
Shenfield GM, Hill JC (1982) Infrequent response by diabetic rats to insulin-liposomes. Clin Exp
    Pharmacol Physiol 9:355–361
Shichiri M, Okada A, Kikkawa R, Kawamori R, Shigeta Y, Abe H (1971) B-Naphthyl-azo-poly-
    styrene-insulin as a means of protecting insulin molecule from digestive enzymes. Biochem
    Biophys Res Comm 44:51–56
Shichiri M, Kawamori R, Yoshida M, Etani N, Hoshi M, Izumi K, Shigeta Y, Abe H (1975)
    Short-term treatment of alloxan-diabetic rats with intrajejunal administration of water-in-
    oil-in-water insulin emulsions. Diabetes 24:971–976
Shichiri M, Kawamori R, Goriya Y, Oji N, Shigeta Y, Abe H (1976) A model for evaluation
    of the peroral insulin therapy: short-term treatment of alloxan diabetic rats with oral water-
    in-oil-in-water insulin emulsions. Endocrinol Jpn 23:493–498
Shichiri M, Yamasaki Y, Kawamori R, Kikuchi M, Hakui N, Abe H (1978) Increased intestinal
    absorption of insulin: an insulin suppository. J Pharm Pharmacol 30:806–808
Shore RN, Shelley WB, Kyle GC (1975) Chronic urticaria from isophane insulin therapy. Sen-
    sitivity associated with noninsulin components in commercial preparations. Arch Dermatol
    111:94–97

Sieber P, Kamber B, Hartmann A, Jöhl A, Riniker B, Rittel W (1974) Totalsynthese von Human-
insulin unter gezielter Bildung der Disulfidbindungen. Helv Chim Acta 57:2617–2621

Sieber P, Kamber B, Hartmann A, Jöhl A, Riniker B, Rittel W (1977) Totalsynthese von Human-
insulin IV. Beschreibung der Endstufen. Helv Chim Acta 60:27–37

Simkin RD, Cole SA, Ozawa H, Magdoff-Fairchild B, Eggena P, Rudko A, Low BW (1970) Precipitation and crystallization of insulin in the presence of lysozyme and salmine. Biochem
Biophys Acta 200:385–394

Slama G, Hautecouverture M, Assan R, Tchobroutsky G (1974) One to five days of continuous
intravenous insulin infusion on seven diabetic patients. Diabetes 23:732–738

Smith DJ, Venable RM, Collins J (1985) Separation and quantitation of insulins and related substances in bulk insulin crystals and in injectables by reversed-phase high performance liquid
chromatography and the effect of temperature on the separation. J Chromatogr Sci 23:81–
88

Smith GD, Swenson DC, Dodson EJ, Dodson GG, Reynolds CD (1984) Structural stability in
the 4-zinc human insulin hexamer. Proc Natl Acad Sci USA 81:7093–7097

Smith KL (1969) Insulin. In: Dorfmann RI (ed) Methods in hormone research vol IIA. Bioassay.
Academic Press, New York, pp 365–414

Steiner DF (1967) Evidence for a precursor in the biosynthesis of insulin. Trans NY Acad Sci
(Ser II) 30:60–68

Steiner DF, Oyer PE (1967) The biosynthesis of insulin and a probable precursor of insulin by
a human islet cell adenoma. Proc Natl Acad Sci USA 57:473–480

Steiner DF, Hallund O, Rubenstein A, Cho S, Bayliss C (1968) Isolation and properties of proinsulin, intermediate forms, and other minor components from crystalline bovine insulin. Diabetes 17:725–736

Stewart GA (1974) Historical review of the analytical control of insulin. Analyst 99:913–928

Stewart WJ, McSweeney SM, Mirle BS, Kellett MA, Faxon DP, Ryan TJ (1984) Increased risk
of severe protamine reactions in NPH insulin-dependent diabetics undergoing cardiac cath-
eterization. Circulation 70:788–792

Storm MC, Dunn MF (1985) The Glu(B13) carboxylates of the insulin hexamer form a cage for
Cd^{2+} and Ca^{2+} ions. Biochemistry 24:1749–1756

Storvick WO, Henry HJ (1968) Effect of storage temperature on stability of commercial insulin
preparations. Diabetes 17:499–502

Strazza S, Hunter R, Walker E, Darnall DW (1985) The thermodynamics of bovine and porcine
insulin and proinsulin association determined by concentration difference spectroscopy.
Arch Biochem Biophys 238:30–42

Strickland EH, Mercola D (1976) Near-ultraviolet tyrosyl circular dichroism of pig insulin
monomers, dimers, and hexamers. Dipole-dipole coupling calculations in the monopole ap-
proximation. Biochemistry 15:3875–3884

Sudmeier JL, Bell SJ, Storm MC, Dunn MF (1981) Cadmium-113 nuclear magnetic resonance
studies of bovine insulin: Two-zinc insulin hexamer specifically binds calcium. Science
212:560–562

Summerell JM, Osmand A, Smith GH (1965) An equilibrium-dialysis study of the binding of zinc
to insulin. Biochem J 95:31P

Sundby F (1962) Separation and characterization of acid-induced insulin transformation products by paper electrophoresis in 7 M urea. J Biol Chem 237:3406–3411

Sutcliffe N, Bristow AF (1984) The proinsulin content of commercial bovine insulin formulations. J Pharm Pharmacol 36:163–166

Szepesi G, Gazdag M (1981) Improved high-performance liquid chromatographic method for
the analysis of insulins and related compounds. J Chromatogr 218:597–602

Tammilehto S, Büchi J (1968) Untersuchungen über die p-Hydroxybenzoesäureester (Nipagi-
ne®). Pharm Acta Helv 43:726–738

Tanford C, Epstein J (1954) The physical chemistry of insulin. I. Hydrogen ion titration curve
of zinc-free insulin. J Am Chem Soc 76:2163–2169

Terabe S, Konaka R, Inouye K (1979) Separation of some polypeptide hormones by high-performance liquid chromatography. J Chromatogr 172:163–177

Thim L, Hansen MT, Norris K, Hoegh I, Boel E, Forstrom J, Ammerer G, Fiil NP (1986) Secretion and processing of insulin precursors in yeast. Proc Natl Acad Sci USA 83:6766–
6770

Thompson EOP, O'Donnell IJ (1960) The chromatography of insulin on DEAE-cellulose in buffers containing 8 M urea. Aust J Biol Sci 13:393–400

Thurow H (1980) Studies on the denaturation of dissolved insulin. In: Brandenburg D, Wollmer A (eds) Insulin chemistry, structure and function of insulin and related hormones. Walther de Gruyter, Berlin New York, pp 215–221

Thurow H, Geisen K (1984) Stabilisation of dissolved proteins against denaturation at hydrophobic interfaces. Diabetologia 27:212–218

Tjioe TO, Wacker A (1972) Reinheitsprüfung von im Handel befindlichen Insulinpräparaten mit Hilfe der diskontinuierlichen Polyacrylamidgel-Elektrophorese. Klin Wochenschr 50:882–884

Touitou E, Donbrow M, Rubenstein A (1980) Effective intestinal absorption of insulin in diabetic rats using a new formulation approach. J Pharm Pharmacol 32:108–110

Tragl KH, Pohl A, Kinast H (1979) Zur peroralen Verabreichung von Insulin mittels Liposomen im Tierversuch. Wien Klin Wochenschr 91:448–451

Trevan JW, Boock E (1962) The standardization of insulin by the determination of the convulsive dose for mice. League of Nations Health III 7:45–56

Tronier B, Larsen UD (1982) Somatostatin-like immunoreactivity in man. Measurement in peripheral plasma. Diabete Metab 8:35–40

Umber F, Störring FK, Föllmer W (1938) Erfolge mit einem neuartigen Depotinsulin ohne Protaminzusatz (Surfen-Insulin). Klin Wochenschr 17:443–446

Unger RH, Aquilar-Parada E, Müller WA, Eisentraut AM (1970) Studies of pancreatic alpha cell function in normal and diabetic subjects. J Clin Invest 49:837–848

United States Pharmacopeia (1980) XX The United States Pharmacopeial Convention, Inc, Rockville. Mack Printing Company, Easton, p 405

Valdenaire K, Klein W (1979) Behandlung von Diabetikern mit Insulinresistenz und -allergie mit Des-Phe-Insulin. Dtsch Med Wochenschr 104:1637–1639

Velcovsky HG, Federlin KF (1984) Experiences in immunological aspects of human insulin. In: Diabetes mellitus: achievements and scepticism. (Royal Society of Medicine International Congress and Symposium Series; no. 77.) Oxford University Press, Oxford, pp 73–81

Vestermark S (1982) Human-Monokomponent (HM)-Insuline in klinischer routinemäßiger Anwendung. Aktuel Endokrinol Stoffwechsel 3:114

Vigneaud V du, Geiling EMK, Eddy CA (1928) Studies on crystalline insulin VI. Further contributions to the question whether or not crystalline insulin is an adsorption product. J Pharmacol Exp Ther 33:497–509

Villalpando S, Drash A (1979) Circulating glucagon antibodies in children who have insulin-dependent diabetes mellitus. Clinical significance and characterization. Diabetes 28:294–299

Vølund Aa, Pingel M, Sørensen E (1982) Differential potency of pork and beef insulins in the USP rabbit bioassay system. In: Gueriguian JL, Bransome ED, Outschoorn AS (eds) Hormone Drugs. United States Pharmacopeial Convention. Rockville, Maryland, pp 208–215

Vontz FK, Puestow EC, Cahill DJ (1982) Anaphylactic shock following protamine administration. Am Surg 48:549–551

Wallhäusser KH (1974) Antimicrobial preservatives in biologics. Pharm Ind 36:716–722

Walters DP, Smith PA, Marteau TM, Brimble A, Borthwick LJ (1985) Experience with NovoPen, an injection device using cartridged insulin, for diabetic patients. Diabetic Medicine 2:490–497

Ward GM, Simpson RW, Ward EA, Turner RC (1981) Comparison of two twice-daily insulin regimens: Ultralente/Soluble and Soluble/Isophane. Diabetologia 21:383–386

Watkins JD, Roberts DE, Williams TF, Martin DA, Coyle V (1967) Observation of medication errors made by diabetic patients in the home. Diabetes 16:882–885

Waugh DF (1946) A fibrous modification of insulin I. The heat precipitate of insulin. J Am Chem Soc 68:247–250

Waugh DF (1948) Regeneration of insulin from insulin fibrils by the action of alkali. J Am Chem Soc 70:1850–1857

Waugh DF (1954) Protein-protein interactions. Adv Protein Chem 9:325–437

Waugh DF (1957) A mechanism for the formation of fibrils from protein molecules. J Cell Comp Physiol (Suppl 1) 49:145–164

Waugh DF, Wilhelmson DF, Commerford SL, Sackler ML (1953) Studies of the nucleation and growth reactions of selected types of insulin fibrils. J Am Chem Soc 75:2592–2600

Weiler JM, Freiman P, Sharath MD, Metzger WJ, Smith JM, Richerson HB, Ballas ZK, Halverson PC, Shulan DJ, Matsuo S, Wilson RL (1985) Serious adverse reactions to protamine sulfate: Are alternatives needed? J Allergy Clin Immunol 75:297–303

Weitzel G, Fretzdorff A-M, Strecker F-J, Roester U (1953) Zinkgehalt und Glukagoneffekt kristallisierter Insulinpräparate. Hoppe-Seyler's Z Physiol Chem 293:190–215

Welinder BS (1980) Gel permeation chromatography of insulin. J Liq Chromatogr 3:1399–1416

Welinder BS (1984) Homogeneity of crystalline insulin estimated by GPC and reversed phase HPLC. In: Hancock WS (ed) CRC Handbook of HPLC for the separation of amino acids, peptides, and proteins, vol II. CRC Press, Inc, Boca Raton, pp 413–419

Welinder BS, Sørensen HH, Hansen B (1986) Reversed-phase high-performance liquid chromatography of insulin. Resolution and recovery in relation to column geometry and buffer components. J Chromatogr 361:357–367

WHO (1980) World Health Organisation. Expert Committee on Diabetes Mellitus. Second Report. Technical Report Series 646, WHO, Geneva, pp 62–63

WHO (1982) World Health Organisation. Expert Committee on Biological Standardization. Technical Report Series 673:29

Wigley FM, Londono JH, Wood SH, Shipp JC, Waldman RH (1971) Insulin across respiratory mucosae by aerosol delivery. Diabetes 20:552–556

Williamson KL, Williams RJP (1979) Conformational analysis by nuclear magnetic resonance: Insulin. Biochemistry 18:5966–5972

Wintersteiner O, Vigneaud V du, Jensen H (1928) Studies on crystalline insulin. V. The distribution of nitrogen in crystalline insulin. J Pharmacol Exp Ther 32:397–411

Yamasaki Y, Shichiri M, Kawamori R, Morishima T, Hakui N, Yagi T, Abe H (1981 a) The effect of rectal administration of insulin on the short-term treatment of alloxan-diabetic dogs. Can J Physiol Pharmacol 59:1–6

Yamasaki Y, Shichiri M, Kawamori R, Kikuchi M, Yagi T, Arai S, Tohdo R, Hakui N, Oji N, Abe H (1981 b) The effectiveness of rectal administration of insulin suppository on normal and diabetic subjects. Diabetes Care 4:454–458

Yip CC, Logothetopoulus J (1969) A specific anti-proinsulin serum and the presence of proinsulin in calf serum. Proc Nat Acad Sci 62:415–419

Yoshida H, Okumura K, Hori R (1979) Absorption of insulin delivered to rabbit trachea using aerosol dosage form. J Pharm Sci 68:670–671

Zeuzem S, Taylor R, Agius L, Schoeffling K, Albisser AM, Alberti KGMM (1985) Biological effects of sulphated insulin in adipocytes and hepatocytes. Mol Cell Biochem 68:161–168

Zoltobrocki M, Enzmann F, Vanderbeke O, Federlin K, Laube H, Klein W, Valdenaire K, Sauer H, Riedesel G, Schöffling K, Neubauer M, Willms B, Ahlhausen M (1980) Erste kontrollierte Multizenterstudie zur Erfassung des Wirkprofils einer neuartigen Insulinzubereitung mit Des-Phe-Insulin (Hoe 03 R = Optisulin Depot). Akt Endokrin 1:41–51

Subject Index